Humanitarian Aid in Post-Soviet Countries

An anthropologist among aid workers. Her objective: to study that exotic tribe, humanitarian and development workers, along with their state and non-state partners, as they 'export democracy' to the post-Soviet countries of Central Asia and the Caucasus. Her method: to join the tribe for ten years. From New York to Alma-Ata, by way of Geneva and Baku, Laëtitia Atlani-Duault provides both an understanding of the individuals working in the field and a critical analysis of the sweeping political implications of NGO activities. A focus on supposedly 'de-politicized' policy areas (notably the prevention of the HIV/AIDS epidemic) provides wider insights into the objectives and practices of international aid workers in countries beset by rising poverty, drug trafficking, prostitution and decaying education and health services. The author also provides a rich canvas of human stories, from the 'workshops' in which diametrically opposed political approaches often clash to the occasional small triumphs in which effective public health interventions are worked out. This timely book will be of great interest not only to scholars of post-Soviet countries, but also to those interested in humanitarian and development aid worldwide. It will also be relevant for the study of the anthropology of development, as well as medical and political anthropology.

Laëtitia Atlani-Duault is Associate Professor (MCF) in Anthropology at the University of Nanterre Paris X (France) and a frequent consultant with humanitarian and development aid agencies in Central Asia and the Caucasus, Eastern Europe and Asia. She is the author of *Au bonheur des autres. Anthropologie de l'aide humanitaire* (Société d'Ethnologie, 2005).

Central Asian Studies Series

Humanitarian Aid in Post-Soviet Countries

An anthropological perspective

Laëtitia Atlani-Duault

Translated by Andrew Wilson

Routledge
Taylor & Francis Group
LONDON AND NEW YORK

First published 2007
by Routledge
2 Park Square, Milton Park, Abingdon, Oxon OX14 4RN

Simultaneously published in the USA and Canada
by Routledge
270 Madison Ave, New York, NY 10016

Routledge is an imprint of the Taylor & Francis Group, an informa business

Typeset in Times New Roman by
Taylor & Francis Books
Printed and bound in Great Britain by
MPG Books Ltd, Bodmin

British Library Cataloguing in Publication Data
A catalogue record for this book is available from the British Library

Library of Congress Cataloging in Publication Data
Atlani-Duault, Laëtitia.
Humanitarian aid in post-Soviet countries : an anthropological perspective / Laëtitia Atlani-Duault.
p. cm. – (Central Asian studies series ; 10)
Includes bibliographical references and index.
1. Humanitarian assistance—Former Soviet republics. 2. Non-governmental organizations—Former Soviet republics. 3. AIDS (Disease)—Former Soviet republics—Prevention. 4. HIV infections—Former Soviet republics—Prevention. I. Title.
HV555.S685A85 2007
362.196'9792009475–dc22 2007022540

ISBN 978-0-415-44884-0 (hbk)
ISBN 978-0-203-93730-3 (ebk)

To Petrev

Contents

Figures

Foreword

Since 1994, I have closely followed Laëtitia Atlani-Duault's work within several international development agencies in New York, Central Asia and the Caucasus.

In this book, she vividly depicts the confrontation that occurred between Soviet and Western models when faced with a shared social phenomenon: the promotion of a development model. She demonstrates that, beyond the question of HIV, it was a confrontation between ways of seeing the world and thinking about collective life. That is where the true strength of this book lies, in its analysis of the political implications of such a confrontation. During the 1990s and particularly after 1992, the principal objective of Westerners in the ex-Soviet Union was to ensure that communism could not return to the region. With this in mind, the development agencies (including mine) dedicated themselves to demolishing the state structures of the Soviet era, as quickly as possible and without viable alternatives to offer. That has caused more social suffering today than ever before. Poverty, drug trafficking, prostitution, a decaying education system and health services, and corruption are major problems in the former Soviet Union after more than ten years of independence. In helping to develop the local non-governmental organization (NGO) sector, the leading development agencies had and gave the impression that local NGOs offered an alternative to the state; there was no thought of them as possible partners in a process of rethinking the role of the state without going as far as dismantling it. Local and international actors participated in these events without always grasping their repercussions, a point this book illustrates with admirable clarity.

Very little material, particularly documented studies, exists on the subject of this book. Most of what has been written about the international development agencies comes from the field of political science. An 'insider' ethnographic approach is completely new. In writing this book, Laëtitia Atlani-Duault has had to work with a great many sceptical government officials, aid agency bureaucrats and self-styled international 'experts' – difficult partners with whom she managed to work with great competence, earning the respect and admiration of all. Critical analysis is always difficult but her insider approach and style of writing have prevailed, resulting in a work that is both understanding of those working in the field and critical of the political implications of their activities. It is a book that should be widely shared.

Ercan Murat

Beginning in 1993, Ercan Murat served as United Nations Resident Representative in a number of countries of Central Asia and the Caucasus. He was also Deputy Director of the UN Development Programme's Regional Office for the former Soviet Union, based in New York, and led the UNDP operations in Afghanistan and Russia. He is now an advisor on international development to UN agencies and other international organizations.

Acknowledgements

This book is not just a translation but a considerable re-working and updating of a book published in French in 2005. I owe a great deal to the many people who have helped me along the way, both with the original book and with this new edition.

First of all, I would like to express my wholehearted thanks to my dear friend and translator, Andrew Wilson, for his work on the English edition of this book. *Merci mille fois*, Andrew.

Special thanks to William Beeman, Rhonda Campbell, Timothy Frasca, Carl Kendall, David Stuart and Benjamin Weil, who reviewed the English edition in depth and took much time to make the manuscript a better book, and to Michael Ames, with all my respect. I am also very grateful to Dorothea Schaefter at Routledge for her support and to the anonymous readers for their helpful comments on an earlier draft of this book.

I would particularly like to express my gratitude to Olivier Herrenschmidt, whose culture and clear thinking have helped this unusual ethnography to take its place within the generalist approach that is fundamental to anthropological research. My gratitude also go to Georges Augustins, Jean-François Baré, Manga Bekombo, Srimoyi Bhattacharya, Doris Bonnet, Jean-François Bouville, Laurence Caillet, Elsa Chabrol, Sophie Cotret, Michèle Cros, Blandine Destremeau, Elisa Escobar, Sophie Houdart, Didier Fassin, Olivier Foulon, Patricia Foxen, François Laplantine, Bruno Lautier, Marc Levy, Jean-Baptiste Martin, Françoise Morin, Ercan Murat, François-René Picon, Catherine Poujol, Jean-Claude Rabier, Richard Rechtman, Cécile Rousseau, Torben Skov, Sandrine Soriano, Boris Sporer, Kristina Tiedje, Laurent Vidal and Zharas Takenov. Without their expertise and their critical and personal involvement, this study would have been very different.

A number of institutions have also financially or materially supported the writing of the book. The work could not have been undertaken without the help of the Laboratoire 'Intervention Publique, Espaces et Sociétés' from l'Institut de Recherche sur le Développement (IRD), the Laboratoire CNRS d'Ethnologie et de Sociologie Comparative (UMR 7535 CNRS-Paris X), the Transcultural Psychiatry Clinic of McGill University / Montreal

Children's Hospital and the Department of Anthropology at Nanterre Paris X University.

Thanks finally to the Atlani and Soyez families. And to Paul, Tom and Mila Duault, for their love.

I dedicate this book to my friends in Central Asia, the Caucasus, New York and Geneva – members of NGOs, governments, international development agencies or common citizens – whose names I cannot include but who are very much present in these pages. It is they who give this research meaning.

Introduction

A day in the 1990s, somewhere along the Caspian Sea. To the visitor, the city's outskirts look like the end of the world. Ruined oil derricks sprawl over miles of flat terrain, some dating back to the Soviet era, others even older, abandoned amidst black lakes of industrial waste. The newest derricks pump lethargically. No vegetation. A persistent, nauseating smell of gas and oil. It is like a lunar landscape or the aftermath of an explosion.

Stuck in the middle of the scene is a 'Detention Centre for Female Prostitutes Infected with Sexually Transmitted Diseases', its sign proclaiming it 'High Priority State Security'. A bunch of mini-vans are parked around the building, their passengers all men in civilian clothes who look more like 'clients' than close relatives of the incarcerated women. The building fits perfectly with its grim surroundings.

Inside, dozens of women, filthy uniforms barely covering their backsides, are watched by male guards. Despite the open windows an unbearable acrid odour is everywhere, a mix of misery and overcrowding. The inmates all have the same look of fear, anger and despair. Given a moment of respite from the guards, they explain that they were too poor to buy off the policemen who stopped them in the street and accused them of prostitution, hoping for 'bakshish' (a bribe). Once accused, they have become enmeshed in the legal system. They come from all over the country.

When will they be freed? 'When the guards and the doctors decide that we are cured. It can take weeks, months, years. There aren't any rules.' Most of them will not return home after they are freed. 'Do you know what it's like to come back from a prison for sick prostitutes?' They end up on the streets of the capital, to which they are strangers.

Two members of the local non-governmental organization (NGO) 'dedicated to the prevention of HIV among imprisoned prostitutes with sexually transmitted diseases' give a detailed factual presentation, graphics included, about the virus and the importance of prevention. The inmates barely pay attention.

The NGO's president, a former journalist, tells me her organization's story in private. Following her first visit to the facility in hopes of writing an article about it, she had been pressured not to report on the abuse she witnessed. Frustrated, but knowing the prison was there to stay, she wanted to do something to help the prisoners. About that time, a major development agency, the International Development Organization (IDO) published a Request-for-Proposal in the newspapers, offering funding for local NGOs active in the field of HIV/AIDS. She answered the advertisement, created her NGO, and her project was chosen by a panel of national and international experts to receive funding. The presentation is part of the new NGO's work in the prevention of HIV.

What makes an international development agency decide to support this type of local NGO? How does it think this will help to 'export democracy'? Can we discern the seeds of the pink, yellow and orange revolutions currently rocking the old Soviet empire?[1]

It is worth remembering that the new post-Soviet states were once integral parts of the USSR, till then the leader of the 'Second World' (Wedel 1996). As the leader of the communist bloc of countries, the USSR was on the same footing as the 'First World', composed of Western countries, and a rival model for a 'Third World' said to be on the road to development. As one observer vividly put it, 'this middle world evaporated in these short five months between the unsuccessful coup against Gorbachev in August 1991 and the end of that year, when the last of the former Soviet republics in Central Asia accepted their independence' (Schoeberlein 2000c: 56). In the historical equivalent of the blink of an eye, these republics not only became independent states but fell from the heights of membership in a great power to the lowly status of developing countries.

When the international development agencies arrived in Central Asia and the Caucasus in the early 1990s there were no local NGOs for the simple reason that the USSR forbade all associations that were independent from official structures. While there were a large number of organizations in each Soviet Republic, any whose activities deviated from the Party or the government 'line' were immediately dissolved. With the demise of the USSR, however, the international development agencies provided massive support for the creation of local NGOs in Central Asia and the Caucasus. This international aid had two foci, one being the promotion of a legal and social framework favouring the creation of local NGOs, and the other being financial and technical assistance for their members. In the name of 'good governance',[2] international organizations were able to help groups of friends or members of former Soviet institutions to create an NGO, register it with the authorities, train its staff, find funding and connect it to international networks. This was so for a wide range of aid and development initiatives, from supporting the creation of private enterprise to fields such as women's rights, education, biodiversity and – this book's particular focus – the prevention of HIV and AIDS. Heterogeneous as they may seem, their common goal was to ensure an environment favourable to 'the emergence and support of local NGOs' and 'the formation of civil society' (Hann 1996, 2002a, 2002b; Wedel 1998).

One might question the reasons for this support, particularly when more than a decade later the pink, orange and yellow revolutions were spearheaded by the same local NGOs, toppling governments inherited from the Soviet era. That is the purpose of this book, the fruit of years working within an international development agency since 1994, both in New York and in the particular, little-studied context of Central Asia and the Caucasus. I will show that this support is part of an institutional ideology, the goal of which, since the beginning of the 1990s, was to create a strong countervailing force against state power and thereby ensure the success of political and economic liberalism in that period of post-Cold War political incertitude.

An anthropology of international aid organizations

The view from inside

Anthropologists working on development phenomena can be divided into two main 'schools', even if the dividing line between applied anthropology and critical anthropology is the subject of numerous debates (Grillo and Stirrat 1997; Hobart 1993; Pottier 1997). The first, the 'applied' anthropology of development, refers to an anthropology focused on practical application, and on providing immediate expertise for development agencies looking to identify, design and improve the implementation of their projects in the field. My study does not fall within the domain of this approach. Indeed, as Didier Fassin puts it, in 'applied' anthropological studies on development,

> we rarely ask an anthropologist to study the cultural world to which he or she belongs, or if we do, it is often to talk about its more exotic aspects. We barely question the thoughts or actions of the political authorities, development officials or doctors, who construct their own representations in terms of knowledge.
>
> (Fassin 1992: 182)

In contrast to practitioners of the applied anthropology of development, who aim to be useful in setting up projects, those associated with the critical anthropology of development do not search for objective 'truths' about development and its effects (Ferguson 1990).[3] They offer critical analysis as much of the implementation of projects as of the epistemological basis on which they stand. They try to understand how the development world is socially constructed and how it constructs its subjects (Escobar 1996).

Three main theoretical approaches are distinguishable in the critical anthropology of development (Olivier de Sardan 2002). The first and oldest approach is a populist one. The study subjects found here are varied, but feature a systematic and often simplistic vaunting of the knowledge of 'the people', an idealized entity, irretrievably poor and oppressed, which needs to be defended (Olivier de Sardan 2002: 729). Robert Chambers" work *Whose Reality Counts? Putting the First Last* (1997), the title of which amply displays his opinion, exemplifies an approach which systematically defends 'small projects versus large ones, appropriate technology versus heavy technology, subsistence culture versus exported cultures, peasant logic and knowledge versus scientific logic and knowledge, rural versus urban, small farmers versus rural entrepreneurs, ... peasant organizations versus big projects, etc.' (Olivier de Sardan 1995: 479).[4]

The second calls on anthropologists to dismantle the development industry's 'discourse'.[5] Arturo Escobar, for example, sees the aim of development projects as instilling among populations the desire for industrial and economic growth, as defined by Western capitalism. Development discourse, according to Escobar, represents the world on a linear scale of progression, on which the North is in the lead and the South is blocked in a static traditionalism that only modern technology and capitalism can transform. Such a 'discourse' stems from neo-colonialism, and acts today as a mechanism for the North's domination of the South (ibid.). It acts as an ideological tool in international relations, with the aim of expanding modern capitalism.

The third approach attempts to avoid both the simplistic over-valuing of folk knowledge and knee-jerk criticism of the 'development business', as well as the over-simple logic of domination versus resistance.[6] In this perspective, rather than considering development as an external force acting on 'real' ethnological field subjects (for example, a given population), recent literature suggests that 'development workers' are themselves valid subjects for fieldwork (Mosse 2005).

Among the still-rare ethnographies trying to examine what is happening in development institutions, two main practices govern choice of field location. The majority of anthropologists have chosen to live among a project's 'beneficiary' population and to follow the trajectory of aid projects from that population's point of view, focusing on the effects of resulting changes on the populations. Their analyses draw their strength from their grounding among the 'beneficiaries' of projects studied. But the development workers themselves remain little studied. Among those who do want to study the 'development worker', however, many do so from the outside.

Reading some of their research, one becomes aware that they have often been working mostly from documents, fleshed out by interviews with development actors, and by observing only some of their practices – those that they are willing to show – forgetting in doing so the research methods of classical anthropology. In some cases, a lack of familiarity with these actors results in fixed and rather simplistic depictions of the mindsets researchers attribute to them. One wonders whether their conclusions about development actors are not heavily influenced by their positions outside the population being studied.

In this study, I have chosen to focus on what we might call a networked ethnography, from within. I emphasize the 'networked' characteristic of this ethnography because the members of a single 'developmentalist configuration'[7] (Olivier de Sardan 1995) do not fit the simple dichotomy of supposedly 'local' populations on one side and 'Western' organizations on the other, as the current stereotype would have it (Grillo and Stirrat 1997; Gupta and Ferguson 1997; Olivier de Sardan 1995; Pottier 1993). In reality, development situations are 'interfaces' not only between field actors, but also between the institutions they represent (some of them multinational) and the representation systems that influence them. As Jean Copans elegantly puts it:

> The development world is not just a universe of networks and of human or financial movements irresistibly enveloping the globe like an ever-expanding ball of wool. It is also a society, a world unto itself of bureaucrats, experts, volunteers and even soldiers who make a living from development but also represent it, socialize it and make it manifest on the ground or in the media.
>
> (Copans 2006:43)

The configuration of actors engaged in IDO's governance and HIV prevention activities in Central Asia and the Caucasus since the collapse of the USSR, is an example (the International Development Organization is one of the most important in the small universe of development agencies, and will be described in greater detail in the following chapter). Note here that the interface is not between New York and village X in Kazakhstan, but between agency representatives – of various nationalities including post-Soviet – and members of the host-country government and local NGOs, who may be based in the ex-USSR, New York or Geneva. One will easily find a German working in Baku, an American in an international agency whose headquarters is in Geneva but who is spending two years in Tashkent, a Belgian dividing his time between Tbilisi and New York, a Kazakh posted to Alma-Ata but trained in Moscow and regularly working at the agency's New York headquarters, or a Kyrgyz based in Bishkek but travelling to multiple international conferences in Europe. These are the types of individual comprising the 'networked' developmental configuration that I am talking about.

Staff working for IDO are divided between headquarters in New York and local offices in so-called developing countries (in Africa, Asia, Latin America and, more recently, East European countries and the ex-USSR). Relations between headquarters and local offices vary. In the majority of cases they are fairly decentralized. Responsibility for field projects falls on the local office, while headquarters handles coordination activities, fundraising, media relations and other concerns. A Resident Representative directs each office. In many multilateral agencies, more than 80 per cent of total staff members currently work in country offices. Most are from the host countries, recruited on site. In Central Asia and the Caucasus, however, local recruitment of IDO employees is relatively recent. Looking to benefit from international assistance to cope with the transition caused by the USSR's collapse, the governments of these newly independent republics requested to be considered by the agencies as potential beneficiaries of assistance, on the same basis as other 'developing' countries (African, Asian, Latin American). One of the first initiatives of these agencies was to open offices in each of these countries. For example, when John arrived in Central Asia in 1993 as the IDO Resident Representative (equivalent to a country bureau chief), he set up his office in a small hotel room, then began negotiations with the government on the conditions of IDO's presence in the country. After several months he transferred his office into a building, furnished it and recruited local staff.

The members of IDO in Central Asia and the Caucasus are therefore not strangers to the region – quite the contrary. In addition, being nationals of one of these countries does not necessarily mean that these actors come from the country. They are not all natives of Turkmenistan even if they have Turkmen nationality, or of Tajikistan if they have Tajik nationality, and so on. One must bear in mind that all these countries were part of the USSR, which was a federation, and that Soviet citizens were deployed across the USSR for reasons that ranged from professional needs to political goals. At the time of the Soviet bloc's collapse and the independence of the countries composing the federation, Soviet citizens acquired a new passport overnight. From being Soviet 'citizens' with multiple 'nationalities', they became Turkmens, Russians or Azeris (Poujol 1993). The allocation of a national passport was not based simply on their place of birth or the number of years spent in a particular region, but also on their place of residence at the time of the collapse of the USSR. Therefore, in the case of three local IDO actors in Kazakhstan, currently Kazakh citizens, the first was born and raised in Yakutia and only settled in Kazakhstan ten years ago, with Soviet citizenship and Jewish 'nationality' (because Jews were considered a 'nationality' during the Soviet era). The second was born and spent part of his childhood in Moscow; the third, born and raised in Kazakhstan during the time of the USSR, was of Korean 'nationality' (large numbers of Koreans were forcibly resettled in Central Asia by the Soviet government during the Korean war). This last one could as easily have been of German origin (the Germans of the Volga were also transferred en masse to Central Asia during the Second World War), Uzbek or Chechen (the Chechens had been deported to Kazakhstan by Stalin and some of them never left). The IDO expatriates were also of different origins and not necessarily from the West, in contrast to the stereotypes often used. A Canadian works alongside a Nepalese, a German and a Zambian. The only thing distinguishing them from the host country nationals is that they do not have the nationality of the country in which they work.

In each country, therefore, the permanent staff of the IDO is composed of local members and expatriates of diverse nationalities who share responsibilities. Staff levels fluctuate according to project needs. When a new aid project is founded, one or several team members are assigned to manage it. They build a team around themselves, made up of external colleagues who are consultants recruited either short term or for the duration of the project. Again, these can be local or foreign. Whatever their origin, these 'development brokers' (Blundo 2000; Olivier de Sardan, Bierschenk and Chauveau 2000) may undertake fixed-term missions, or remain for years in the field. In addition, depending on the projects, the IDO staff will work in close collaboration with members of governments, local NGOs, village representatives, the media or even local businesses.

In addition to these networked activities, these staff members on the whole move easily from one post to another. A member of a local NGO, for example, may well be recruited by an international NGO, or by an international development agency, whether in his/her own country or in a foreign land. One might also see a European university professor taking several years off to work with local communities and help them create their own network in response to development projects, while another provides his/her expertise to a large international development bank in the same country. An activist from an international NGO may equally be recruited by an international development agency to work as an expatriate expert in a foreign country, as in the case of Mike, whom we will soon meet.

Government representatives also move just as frequently from one post to another, trading for example a government bureau for a local NGO delegation – like Tatiana, one of the characters in this study – or a post within an international development agency. We come to understand that it is impossible to assume that actors belong within certain categories with known and fixed characteristics, determined entirely by nationality or affiliation to a particular institution at any given time. It would certainly be simplistic to say that all the IDO representatives, for example, dedicate themselves to proselytizing, like 'Western missionaries'. The dichotomy of locals and internationals, or NGOs and international development agencies, is inadequate to help one understand the development world's discourse and practice in the field. Developmental configurations function as networks and must be understood as such.

The way to undertake an 'insider' ethnography and study an international ideology under construction is both to carry out a 'multi-situated ethnography' (Marcus 1995; Marcus 1998; Burawoy *et al.* 2000), and to participate as fully as possible in the community being studied (Bellier and Wilson 2000). The latter means trying to blend in with the group and become like them – in my case, to become like my colleagues Mike, Beth or John, whom we come across in these pages. I wanted to understand the underlying logic of the actors' choices, the activities they develop, the representations woven and the gaps between principle and practice (Ferguson 1990). Doing so took me years of work and research (from 1994 to 2003) in Central Asia, in the Caucasus, in New York and in Geneva, complemented by periodic working missions to the field. During those years, I found acceptance among the teams of IDO 'development workers'. To begin with (in 1994), I applied for an internship. Very soon, I was working in a full-time job. For nearly ten years my work consisted of listening, studying, observing, reading and writing internal documents, helping people to outline and describe their work, their backgrounds, their bright ideas and annoyances, and their achievements. This was a privileged position from which to carry out my study, because to understand my colleagues and help them articulate their work and thoughts in terms with which they were comfortable, I needed to spend time with them, understand their points of reference, their surroundings, their writings, their activities, and to bring to the surface whatever it was they wanted me to help them understand – and in doing so, to access, at their request, a thorough understanding of their universe.[8] The same people regularly asked me to work with them, and recommended me to their colleagues, which is how I was able to follow the same projects and the same teams over a number of years.

When the possibility of undertaking ethnographical studies on actors in the development field is brought up, the usual criticisms arise which highlight the difficulty of being accepted within the institutions. As J.F. Baré notes,

> we sometimes object that their approach is not an easy one and especially that political-administrative structures are closed and guarded worlds. We agree, but must remember that investigating the genealogy of a Madagascan peasant is not easily undertaken either. In the case of administrative officers, exactly as in the case of Madagascan peasants, one must create for oneself a common communication zone which allows the interlocutor to recognize himself in the interview. In both cases, therefore, it is a question of approach, the ability to create and maintain a certain confidence, and not a question of the subject under study. … It all depends on the researcher's capacity to generate confidence.
>
> (2001: 111–13)

My position was occasionally the source of questions; at the same time as I took part in this collective effort, in which I shared both the work and the risks, I also had to distance myself to act as an observer. But while this could a priori have seemed a contradiction inherent in being both actor and observer, it was never a source of misunderstanding with international or local partners, agency staff, local NGOs, government representatives or participants in the activities I have described. In fact, it would be simplistic to believe that, because they are actors, they would not be critical, sometimes passionately, of their practices, or that they would avoid thinking about the hidden or manifest risks of their missions in order not to see the full effects of their work. Each development worker is to some degree both observer and actor. The critical analysis set forth here does not aim to devalue in any way the importance of the work accomplished on behalf of persons affected by HIV/AIDS in the region, but to thoroughly understand the political mechanisms linked to any and all institutional approaches to development aid.

It would certainly have been easier to opt for a different approach, one far more widely used in this type of study, which would have omitted all mention of my dual status as both actor (I participated, like my colleagues, on behalf of an international development organization in activities which I describe later in the book) and observer (it was in my own work and my relations with my interlocutors that I found the raw material used to critically analyse this complex group's professional practice, which translated de facto into a given policy for development aid). It would have been perfectly possible to not 'expose' my dual position, to leave myself out when recounting the work and thinking processes of the other actors – maintaining the scholar's comfortable exemption from contradiction, enjoying total freedom of observation, participating but never engaging and therefore never having to question the justice, assumptions and appropriateness of what I was doing, never being forced to separate out what I knew, what I did, what I was meant to do and what I was meant to think.

Leaving myself out of the group of actors described here would also have been to submit to the dictum that one cannot be both actor and observer without one of these roles undermining the other, just as one cannot both knead dough and keep one's hands clean. But I reject this timorous and mistaken vision. I affirm the indivisibility of knowledge and action, of knowing and doing, of theoretical knowledge and technical competence. I openly acknowledge in these pages my position of observer and actor, as I did in the field with my partners, as engaged as any of them in the situations and processes studied. Affirming my dual role honours the richness of the human relations established with the actors in the field during the course of the research, as well as declaring my interest. I may therefore declare my real esteem and (for the most part) profound sympathy for a group of impressive and hardworking individuals, without in any way restricting the necessary critique of the political ideologies underpinning some of their actions.

This position emphasizes that without the day-to-day work and effort of thousands of people – from international development agencies such as IDO, local NGOs and governments, and various actors involved in the fight against HIV/AIDS that we will come across in these pages – the impact of the epidemic would be far more devastating, in this region as elsewhere.

To some extent, the book was written in order to make more widely known the importance of the efforts by international development agencies like IDO and its non-governmental partners. If that means calling some aspects of these efforts into question, it is done with the intention of helping to improve them

A shifting 'institutional ideology'

Finally, because the actors in my study were working in the field of HIV/AIDS prevention, I needed methodological tools that would dig beneath the smoothed-out, politically correct and technocratic superficialities of discourse on HIV/AIDS in the development world, and grasp their political coherence. I found them not in the anthropological literature of development, but in the literature of medical anthropology on AIDS. Authors such as Peter Aggleton, Dennis Altman, Tony Barnett, Gilles Bibeau, Jean-Pierre Dozon, Gary Dowsett, Laurent Vidal, Paul Farmer, Didier Fassin, Susan Hunter, Shirley Lindenbaum, Merrill Singer, Carl Kendall and Richard Parker, to cite only a few among many, address the social, political and economic conditions in which medical science on HIV and AIDS is produced. They show that many actors in the field of health tend to present their views and practices as if they have a purely scientific basis, which is historically, culturally and politically neutral.

I was also inspired by Allan Young's study of the notion of 'post-traumatic stress disorder'. In this study (1995), Young takes the ethnography of a diagnostic definition, post-traumatic stress disorder, from the psychiatric classification system standardized by the American Association of Psychiatry in the *Diagnostic and Statistical Manual of Mental Disorders*. The adoption of this manual is part of a revolution in thinking and acting that took place within North American psychiatry in the late 1960s. Through ethnography from within psychiatric institutions, Young found a genealogy of ideas which led to the creation and adoption, by the Western psychiatric community, of this new thinking on the set of mental problems that make up the notion of post-traumatic stress disorder.

What interests me here is what Young calls an 'institutional ideology', a notion that we borrow to delimit our study focus. As he notes,

> I am writing about an institutional ideology, and not a pervasive, society-wide set of ideas. I call the ideology's beliefs and practices 'ideological' because (1) they are used to convince people to do things they might otherwise not want to do, (2) they subvert or devalue critical ideas that might lead people to behave in other ways, and (3) they serve important interests, as identified by the Institute's directors, by either transforming or overwhelming resistances in the mandated production process. Put into other words, this ideology is a medium that ensures the Institute's knowledge producers are integrated in the detailed division of labour.
> (1995: 116)

'Not every institution necessarily has an ideology', remarks Young:

> In some institutions, power holders have effective ways of controlling people through surveillance, coercion, and rewards, and ideologies are

> not needed to convince people to behave correctly. In other institutions, ideology is superfluous because power is shared, technical knowledge is evenly distributed, and labour power, skills, motivation, technology and modes of social organization are sufficient for meeting institutional goals and individual and collective want.
>
> (1995: 116)

In the international development agencies, an institutional ideology is necessary for two main reasons: because there is no tight control of staff members working in 'developing countries', and because an ideology must be constantly justified within a given institution as well as externally. It is moreover this necessity of constant justification which permits us to follow the complicated pathways of forming an institutional ideology. To hear them talk, development workers often seem to have adopted whole the latest 'result' of their institutional ideology's ongoing construction. In doing so, they often forget the 'result's' links back to its origin, despite that being essential to understanding the logic underpinning their practices and ideas.

Studying the construction of IDO's institutional ideology of good governance was not easy. In reality, the process of creating norms and legitimizing practices is done bit by bit as the actors involved (foreigners and locals, university scholars and international bureaucrats, members of local NGOs, *apparatchiks*, representatives of donor countries and people living with HIV/AIDS) work together, get on, quarrel, like each other, detest each other, see their friends and relatives fall ill, see others get ahead. Discourse and practice are intertwined (Apthorpe and Gasper 1996). The first is constructed through the second, while the second feeds on the first. Following this construction therefore means following years of internal debate, opposition, changes of direction, reversal of positions and the causes of such reversals, and issues that are never questioned and the reasons behind their apparent indisputability (Latour 1987, 1993, 1999). It means searching out the roots of these constructions as they spring from the complexity of life in the field, from contradictory explanations, false starts and shortcuts, all of which suddenly take form and link together (Laplantine 2003). This is particularly difficult within international development agencies such as IDO, where debates are played out in the corridors, in small groups, by email, during conferences or workshops in scattered countries, and through grey literature.[9] The institution does not maintain a precise institutional memory. That is neither its goal nor its concern. On the contrary – as we shall see.

Dialogue and debate

This book is divided into four chapters. They present an ethnological study of the successive stages in the construction of the institutional ideology in all its debates, detours and adaptations.

Part of the ethnographic material takes the form of dialogues, based on my notes. I have included these debates in the text because such discussions are an integral part of the reality of development projects. It is through debate between various actors that institutional ideology is defined, shaped, critiqued, modified and reshaped. The source of much of an organization's discourse and operational practice, these debates also constitute a field in which an ethnologist can gather data. All through the book the reader will come across a development agency that I have named the International Development Organization (IDO); local NGOs such as Boda, Sisao, Narco, the Dynamic Youth NGO and the NGO of Active Women; expatriates or IDO local staff such as Igor, Mike, Beth, John and Anna; Olozbiek, the head of public health in an isolated *oblast*; Vladimir and Eldar, both of them secretaries of state for AIDS in their respective Ministries of Health; Lena, formerly Vladimir's assistant at the state secretariat; and members of local NGOs such as Tatiana, Alexey, Atkan, Slava and Piotr. While these organizations and persons accurately reflect the information I gathered about real institutions and existing individuals, they should not be treated by the reader as specific organizations or individuals but as representative types. In order that the actors and their institutions remain anonymous, names and physical attributes have been changed; some of those mentioned are amalgams of several people. Many of the events described have been disguised as to time and place, and the names of the countries in which they occurred are not identified.

Over the years I formed bonds of familiarity with a number of them. They supported me not only in my collection of data but also during times of doubt, fear and illness. It was they, along with my anthropologist friends, who convinced me to continue the research, to keep on collecting fragments of experience for analysis. Their confidence also allowed me to overcome the ambivalence that Philippe Bourgeois – like other ethnologists – experienced during his research in Harlem in the early 1990s. As he noted, 'most ethnologists display a certain empathy with the culture or the people they study. … Ethnologists never want to give their subjects an unattractive image. One must make presentable those that are vulnerable' (Bourgeois 1995: 43). It seems to me essential, from both an ethical and analytical point of view, to describe the varied realities of the development experience in this region as accurately as possible, while avoiding a voyeuristic emphasis on violence or corruption which would comfortably fit with currently fashionable anti-Soviet and anti-agency stereotypes. Breaching their anonymity would be a betrayal of their confidence in me. I would also be putting myself in danger if I return to the region: during my fieldwork, I received several warnings, notably an abortive kidnapping at gunpoint – which certain highly experienced colleagues interpreted as a 'message' for me to keep silent on my findings. For this is a region, let us remember, which is the theatre of conflicts linked with petroleum interests and corruption, and a major route for drug trafficking.

1 The first steps

Since the early 1990s, the idea of 'exporting democracy' under the guise of 'good governance' has been the major point of reference for the work of international agencies in developing countries. It is not limited to theory but amounts to a major social phenomenon. In its name, thousands of people are employed, hundreds of millions of dollars are channelled each year to 'developing' countries, local and international realities are transformed. What is this governance which, since the mid-1990s, has become a central element of political expression at international and national levels, and indeed is used to guide the functioning of authority in large companies? Official texts at the United Nations and the World Bank, among other international institutions, try to give it a practical definition. This supposedly new notion denotes 'an economic, political and administrative exercise with the aim of managing a country's affairs at every level' (UNDP 1998: 3) and over the last ten years a substantial corpus of guidelines has been developed in its name by the major international development agencies.[1]

At the heart of this new body of work, the aim of the international agencies is to aid local NGOs in developing countries on the grounds that NGOs are (supposedly) representative of civil society and provide a counterbalance to the power of governments. Assistance to local NGOs, perceived as a guarantee of good governance, is now accepted by bilateral (e.g., USAID) and multilateral organizations (the World Bank, UNICEF, the United Nations Development Programme (UNDP), the World Health Organization (WHO), and others) as relevant to what they see as a new ethics of development.

Supporting local NGOs rather than the state may seem paradoxical: development agencies are the creation of governments and need the agreement of a given country's government before they can establish their aid projects there. This characteristic is the basis of much criticism of these agencies, accused of being 'in the pockets' of governments. Supporting local NGOs within a framework of promoting good governance may, in addition, be the latest manifestation of an older concern with supporting the ownership of projects by the populations concerned. A talisman of international development organizations, this preoccupation has actually taken many forms during the past few decades, such as the struggle for 'participation' of local actors as part of their self-development, and respect for their 'traditions'.

It would seem, however, that the meaning and practices surrounding the notion of good governance actually stem from a new 'humanitarian ideology' rising from the ruins of Third World-ism. To analyse it, I chose to look at a specific area of this supposedly universal support for good governance in countries of the South, newly expanded towards the East: the area of HIV prevention. There are two reasons for this choice. The first is that this epidemic is both a revealing indicator and a factor of social change for modern societies. The second reason is that the NGOs involved in the fight against the HIV/AIDS epidemic in North America and Europe are often engaged in all sorts of battles around sexuality, inequality of the sexes, the pharmaceutical industry, the politics of the market or public health reform. The policy of good governance encourages development agencies to present this phenomenon as typical of the involvement of local NGOs.

New York, New York

This story begins during the winter of 1994 in New York, on the seventh floor of the International Development Organization (IDO) headquarters. It is a composite world, partly a mirror of American big city life but also a specific environment where actors' behaviour is set against the norms and culture of an international institution. I came originally for a short-term internship that soon turned into a fixed-term post, spending over a year in the office that oversees development aid in countries of the former USSR.

In line with New York corporate lifestyle everyone's place in IDO's hierarchy was discernible by the office space allocated to them. For the Chiefs, an office with outward-facing windows, the number of windows being in direct proportion to the hierarchical status of the beneficiary; for others, an office with artificial lighting facing the corridor. During my first few days, confined to a cubicle, I began to have problems with my eyesight. Worried, I consulted an ophthalmologist, and requested office space with natural daylight. I was given one, but in the process attracted considerable hostility from an Assistant Chief who had waited years before obtaining such a 'privilege'. This hostility took a while for me to understand. A few months later, less naïve, I noticed a team of building maintenance workers in the corridors, and this time immediately understood what was going on: they had come to shift the dividing walls between two offices which until then had been of similar size, each one having two windows. The occupant of the office on the left had recently been promoted and therefore merited three windows; hence the repositioning of the dividing wall, taking one of the windows from her now lower-ranked neighbour to the right.

The institution

Created after the Second World War, IDO is one of the world's largest development agencies. Its goal is to help developing countries to eliminate poverty, to preserve and regenerate the environment and to empower people and institutions. In the mid-1990s, when this book begins, the focus of the organization was on the fight against poverty and on community participation. In both of these areas, the emphasis was on strengthening national capacity, itself part of an overall approach of 'sustainable development'.

IDO is financed by voluntary annual contributions. Its principal donors, depending on the year, are the USA, Japan, Denmark, the Netherlands, Germany, Norway, Sweden, France, the United Kingdom, Canada, Switzerland, Italy, Belgium, Austria, Australia, Finland and Spain. An internationally agreed-upon procedure determines the level of contribution by beneficiary countries to normal operations, taking into consideration each country's population and per capita gross national product (GNP). Other criteria apply to countries with significant geographical handicaps or major economic difficulties.

IDO's defining activities – the transfer of knowledge and the funding of development – have existed since well before the organization was created. In the colonial era, this approach to stimulating markets within colonies was a means of reinforcing the metropolitan economy. However, the real processes of transferring knowledge and financing development aid began at the end of the Second World War. The International Monetary Fund (IMF) and the International Bank for Reconstruction and Development (IBRD, better known as the World Bank) were founded at the Bretton Woods Conference in 1944, and were followed by the FAO (Food and Agriculture Organization) in 1945. Unlike bilateral aid, which is the transfer of funds from one government to another, multilateral aid comprises many donors acting as one, with no single donor directly controlling the aid programme.

At the same time, numerous bilateral agencies were created by the wealthiest nations. These include France's Ministry of Cooperation, the United States Agency for International Development (USAID, created in 1961), the German Agency for Technical Cooperation (*Deutsche Gesellschaft für technische Zusammenarbeit*, or GTZ) and its British equivalent (the Department for International Development, DFID). International non-governmental organizations (NGOs) active in development aid were also set up. Alongside the latter emerged local or national NGOs operating only in their country of origin. For example, an NGO created by a Bangladeshi citizen to help the women of Bangladesh create small businesses through micro-credit is categorized as national or local, so long as its activities do not go beyond the boundaries of Bangladesh (Ryfman 2004).

Various organizational actors in the development world created projects or programmes,[2] and set about defining the methods and beneficiaries,[3] as we shall see (Figure 1.1).

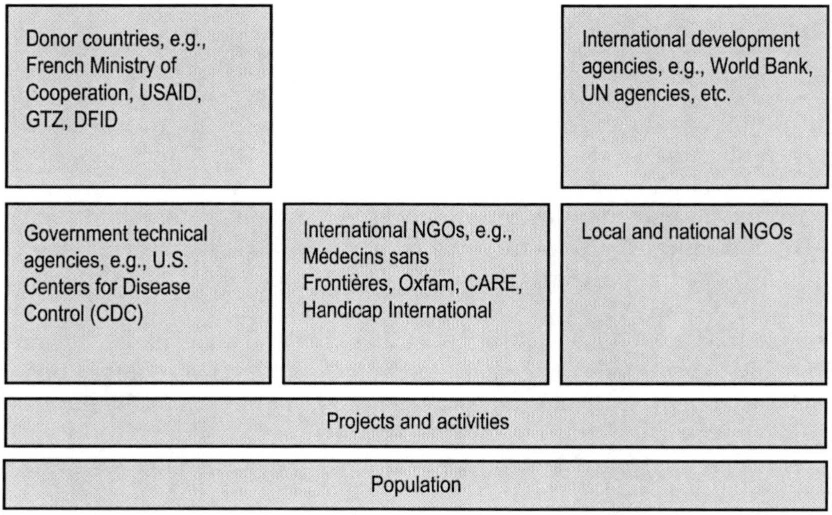

Figure 1.1 Financial flows and potential partnerships between different types of development agencies (based on Gardner and Lewis 1996: 9).

The field

Through a network of more than one hundred international offices, the IDO works in almost two hundred countries and territories in Africa, Asia and the Pacific, Latin America and the Caribbean, the Arab States, Eastern Europe and the ex-USSR. As the decentralized operational arm of IDO, this network of local offices provides various services, from supporting the creation of development programmes with policy advice to practical development work at country level. As we will see, the local offices constitute an information exchange network on a global scale, and provide ongoing training in development both to government employees and to the staff of IDO and their local partners. More than 80 per cent of IDO's employees work in these country offices, and a similar proportion of staff in these offices are nationals of the host countries, recruited on site.

IDO staff members are thus divided between headquarters in New York and the local offices in developing countries. Reporting relationships between headquarters and local offices vary, but normally there is a certain amount of decentralization. Responsibility for field-based projects falls to the local office, while such tasks as coordination of activities, monitoring and evaluation, fundraising, reporting to donors and media relations are handled by headquarters. The New York headquarters is made up of several departments, including regional offices that cover the agency's development programmes in each major region of the world. There are regional offices for Africa, Asia, Latin America and the Caribbean, the Arab states, and finally an office created in the early 1990s for the countries of the ex-USSR and Eastern Europe.

All IDO local offices are run by National Representatives. In the interests of efficiency and decentralization, they are authorized to approve substantial budget projects on their own. Approval from New York is only necessary when project budgets exceed a particular threshold, or concern more than one country. The latter are called regional projects, and are often managed by headquarters, that is by the regional offices or the technical specialized offices. At the top of the hierarchical pyramid, National Representatives and New York offices are supervised by the Executive Head, who answers to a Programme Board.

In each IDO regional office, the programme managers direct the organization's activities, following standardized codes of management. One manager may be given responsibility for creating and implementing activities focused on women, another for micro-credit programmes, a third for the organization of elections. Managers are based in New York, undertaking numerous missions to those countries affected by the activities for which they are responsible. Nevertheless, the IDO regional office in charge of ex-USSR and Eastern European countries in 1994 is not comparable in any degree with the other regional offices of the organization. It still has few personnel and budgets are small because the countries of the former Soviet Union have only very recently come to be considered developing countries, having thus lost their rank – and their privileges – as contributors to the organization's budget. Among African, Latin American and Asian countries that have been classed as 'developing' for a long period of time, many grumble about the fact that IDO largesse must now be shared with these newcomers.

The regional office for Eastern Europe and the former Soviet Union has little specific knowledge of the region because until very recently it was one of the great world powers, and therefore unlikely to receive development aid. The majority of staff, like my colleagues Beth, Anna, Mike or John (whom you will meet in the following chapters), are development professionals with experience working in Africa, Asia and Latin America, and know little or nothing about the ex-USSR.[4] As will be seen, they gradually come to understand that the analyses, concepts and methods used in the 'Third World' for decades are ill adapted to the 'Second World' of the former Soviet republics.

A very small minority of the members of the New York team come from the ex-USSR. There are a few old *apparatchiki* who were employed by their governments during the Soviet era. Shaped by Soviet work practices, in 1994 they have little understanding of the agency's internal functioning or more generally of the development field. There are also some under-30s, who did not work for their governments during the Soviet era, but who are often from the intellectual and political elite of their countries. This has given them the opportunity to acquire a perfect command of foreign languages and the ability to integrate rapidly into the United States-based international agencies. Although they are personally well acquainted with the region, they have no training in development issues and little previous professional experience to call on. For them, it is a time to invent, pioneer, innovate and even improvise. One needs to know how to take the initiative, persuade, define an action programme and find the funding.

Paradigm change: the development of 'development'

The story begins at a moment when IDO already has thirty years of international experience. To understand how the various actors will create new methods for the promotion of good governance through activities such as HIV prevention that are, at first glance, unrelated, we need a brief genealogy of the ideas constituting the theoretical 'building blocks' current in New York at the beginning of our story.

In the mid-1960s, when IDO was created, the dominant hypothesis of the development paradigm was that economic growth – measured by economic indices such as GNP or per capita income – would result in a general rise in the standard of living thanks to the 'trickle-down effect', which would tend to reduce poverty (Copans 2006). This dominant theme among development professionals held that there was an inverse relationship between redistribution policies and growth. This was based on a simple principle: redistributing the income of the rich to the less rich would cause a reduction in the level of savings and thus reduce the economy's rate of growth. This paradigm of modernization also anticipated that incomes would tend to automatically equalize if growth was fast enough to use up excess manpower. It was usually assumed that this would automatically lead to positive changes in other indices, such as rates of infant mortality and so on.

> Even if not everyone benefits directly from growth, the 'trickle-down-effect' will ensure that the riches of those at the top of the economic scale will eventually benefit the rest of society through increased production and thus employment. . . . Development is quantifiable and thus reducible to economics.
>
> (Gardner and Lewis 1996: 7)

In this framework, development aid was conceived as technical assistance aiming to increase the economic growth of poor countries. Development in these countries varied according to their position on a graduated scale of pre-determined stages of economic growth (Rostow 1960). In such a context, IDO's development aid in the 1960s focused chiefly on the creation of industries and urban infrastructure. Large-scale industrialization was considered the basis of economic growth, itself the long-term guarantor of reduced inequalities between rich and poor countries (Ferguson 1999). Democracy was supposed to follow. Although the paradigm of modernization tended to concentrate aid in urban zones, the agency also took an interest, albeit to a lesser extent, in rural areas, following the example of other development agencies at that time. This was particularly true during the 'green revolution' when agriculture received special attention, and which led to a significant increase in food production in some countries.[5] In both urban and rural zones, IDO's favoured partner was the state, which was assumed to bear the entire responsibility for the reforms and essential investments needed to bring about economic growth and social well being.

Little critiqued until the end of the 1960s and the beginning of the 1970s, this paradigm of modernization began to show serious flaws. The economic gap between rich and poor countries increased. Cases where technological changes were associated with greater inequality and the collapse of traditional mutual assistance networks began to be commonplace. The international political economy was also changing. Petroleum crises, the liberalization of finances, and the weight of the Cold War contributed to the emergence of a new perspective in the way that development professionals, those of IDO included, thought about development. This new perspective was heavily influenced by neo-Marxist theory, which led to numerous debates on development in the 1970s. From this perspective, capitalism being inherently unequal, economic growth means that some parts of the world and some social groups are actively underdeveloped (Frank A. Gunder 1992).[6] Even though the paradigm of modernization continued to dominate thinking among development experts, the new perspective – understood to be based in macro and micro inequalities – became widely held in the 1970s, and in certain circles up until the 1980s. That may be linked to what would become the focus on 'basic needs' made popular by the International Labour Organization, which emphasized the fight against poverty and the 'participation of local communities', rather than the promotion of industrialization and modernization. It said that the work of development ought to be centred on eliminating poverty, with the main goal of meeting the primary needs of populations.[7] Adopting this new perspective, IDO reoriented its priorities and re-centred itself around actions aimed at creating employment, providing food for all, and improving health, education and social services for the most needy, as well as a better redistribution of income.

For many, however, this new outlook did not fundamentally address the above assumptions, 'but instead involved an amended agenda in which vulnerable groups such as "small farmers" or "women-headed households" were targeted for aid. Many of these projects were strongly welfare-oriented and did not challenge existing political structures' (Gardner and Lewis 1996: 7). So although 'community participation' had much greater emphasis than before, the state remained the privileged interlocutor of development agencies in developing countries (Copans 2006).

At the end of the 1970s and the beginning of the 1980s, the slowing of world growth, the burden of debt (particularly in Latin America and Africa), a succession of natural disasters and an increase in international instability, led – unevenly of course – to mediocre economic performances in many developing countries. This resulted in a questioning of development aid funding. A major criticism of current development policies was that the 'trickle-down effect', so highly praised, in fact rarely existed (Copans 2006). It was clear that growth – and even meeting the 'basic needs' of the most vulnerable populations – did not lead directly to improved conditions for populations as a whole. 'As societies in the affluent North demonstrate, the increased use of highly sophisticated technology or a fast-growing GNP does not necessarily eradicate poverty, illiteracy or homelessness, although it may well alter the ways these ills are experienced' (Gardner and Lewis 1996: 7).

In addition, the optimism of the 1960s and early 1970s, when many newly independent small states experienced economic growth, was replaced by growing pessimism in the 1980s. This was particularly true in Africa and Latin America where populations were faced with substantial debt, unequal relations of international trade, and, in a number of cases, political instability. The role of the state was thrown into question and some state economic policies were criticized as being too interventionist.

The rise of 'sustainability'

From the mid-1980s, stabilization regimes and structural adjustment programmes implemented by the World Bank and the International Monetary Fund occupied centre stage, and many governments were forced to accept them. The objective of the international financial institutions was to help developing countries respond to economic crises of the time. The recommended measures aimed to re-establish macroeconomic balances and to find (or get back to) the path to growth. The accent was placed on economic performance and the need to reduce government intervention in the market. A number of countries undertook structural adjustment programmes targeting market deregulation, a less interventionist state apparatus, limits on salary increases, reduced public expenditure, privatization, freeing of prices, and free circulation of capital. Moreover, the international agencies reviewed the role assigned to the state in development policies. While this was going on, the work of some development agencies such as IDO and UNICEF remained centred on fighting poverty and the causes of under-development.[8] But they no longer demanded that the state act as the all-powerful provider of economic and social growth in developing countries. On the contrary, it was expected that the state would limit its role to that of a 'catalyst' and a 'facilitator' (to use the vocabulary of the time) of economic reforms.

Contrary to expectation, the impact of structural adjustment programmes on the populations of many countries was disastrous. At the end of the 1980s and the beginning of the 1990s it became clear that they had had a phenomenal economic and social cost. Although formerly considered the only remedy which would allow these countries to enter into a virtuous cycle of development, structural adjustment programmes now became regarded as only one instrument among many others (Muet 1993). Redistribution policies and reduction of inequalities as elements in economic growth took on a higher profile, along with 'safety net' social policies to absorb the shock of adjustment.

Two key moments marked this evolution. The first was the 1992 Earth Summit in Rio de Janeiro, organized by the United Nations. Rio contributed greatly to making it understood that the environment and development are closely linked, an idea underpinning the notion of 'sustainable development'. The latter term appeared in the Brundtland report (World Commission on Environment and Development 1987) which defined it as 'development that meets the needs of the present without compromising the ability of future generations to meet their own needs'. In an oft-cited reference, the economist Robert Solow (1993) formulated the term in a more precise way as 'an obligation to conduct ourselves so that we leave the future the option or the capacity to be as well off as we are'. From this foundation, each international organization went on to define what it understood by sustainable development. For IDO it was an increase in the choices offered to all people making up society, thereby putting men and women – particularly the poor and the vulnerable – at the centre of development processes. The expression also included protection of future generations' options and 'the natural systems on which all forms of life depend'.

With this new objective in mind, and not solely the criteria of economic growth and per capita income, the impact of former development policies was critically re-evaluated. For example, the *World Report on Human Development*, published later on in 1996 by the United Nations Development Programme (UNDP), provided evidence that economic growth does not automatically lead to sustainable human development or the elimination of poverty. In fact, countries which rank high based on per capita income often rank lower if the indicator of human development is used. It also showed that there were strong disparities within countries – rich or poor – often at the expense of native populations and ethnic minorities. As a result, international development agencies, including IDO, increasingly adapted their development policies according to the new approach of the links between growth and poverty.

The rise of 'governance'

The second key moment in this evolution was the publication in 1989 of a World Bank report which caused a great deal of discussion (World Bank 1989).

In its analysis of the increase in poverty and under-development in sub-Saharan Africa, this report stated that one of the major factors explaining the failure of development policies in the region was a crisis of 'governance'. This was the first use of the word in the field of international development.

It appeared in an assessment – mostly negative – of structural adjustment policies implemented during the 1980s, which recommended better control of reform measures (Osmont 1998).

> The necessity of structural adjustment being ever more pressing, it was absolutely essential that economic reforms be strengthened in the areas of norms and regulation/deregulation, but also in public finance, administration, and the civil service. This required fighting corruption, transparency of budget decisions, and reorganizing both public services and, ultimately, the form [mode] of government.
>
> (Osmont 1998: 19)

The Bank came to define the term as 'the manner in which power is exercised ... in the management of a country's social and economic reforms' (World Bank 1992).[9]

Little by little, although still very vaguely defined in 1989, the term took root in the discourse of international development agencies. By the second half of the 1990s there was no getting away from it, as the majority of international development agencies had adopted the term (Smouts 1998). For example, UNDP used it for the first time in a document in 1992; its use became common within the organization by 1995 and system-wide by 1997. UNDP defined it as:

> the exercise of economic, political and administrative authority to manage a country's affairs at all levels. It comprises the mechanisms, processes and institutions through which citizens and groups articulate their interests, exercise their legal rights, meet their obligations and mediate their differences.
>
> (UNDP 1997c: 4)

Beyond such basic definitions (which varied between agencies), a veritable corpus of moral guidelines was developed in the name of good governance during the 1990s. With the uncertainty sparked by the fall of the Berlin Wall and emergence of a multi-polar world, new normative landmarks were needed (Rosenau and Czempiel 1992; Smouts 1998). The World Bank's promotion of good governance was thus not only a policy driven by political objectives but also 'a mode of government in Foucault's sense' (Lautier 2001: 170).

With this new corpus of guidelines, the 'myth of the state' of the 1960s – which had itself been replaced in the 1980s by the 'myth of the state and the market' – morphed yet again into 'the myth of the state, the market and civil society' (Humes and Edward 1997). Despite the diversity of forms covered by the generic term non-governmental organization, and despite its ambiguity (see for example Deler *et al.* 1998; Pratt 2003; Ryfman 2004), the NGOs of the South are generally held to be archetypal manifestations of this vaguely defined civil society. The reality is that although they figured for years in the rhetoric of community mobilization, the NGOs of the South had been relatively marginalized in development policies, compared to the emphasis given the state and the market. Today, however, the international agencies seem to be giving them new functions as part of the good governance agenda, a transformation based on two principles.

The first concerns the balance between state, markets and NGOs. The market and private enterprise are considered the most efficient mechanisms for both 'democratizing' and 'developing' a country. Privatization of public services and institutions is recommended, along with anything that does not need the authority of state power to function (Peters and Pierre 1998; Stoker 1998: 19). The state is no longer considered the principal actor in public management, and must share its responsibilities with the private sector and the non-governmental sector (Lachapelle and Paquin 2004; Laroche 2003). From this perspective, the international agencies are supposed to support the activities of Southern NGOs as they take charge of public goods and services in what might be called a social market (Clayton 1997a, 1997b; Weiss and Gordenker 1996). Although these NGOs have been supported for many years by the agencies, they now seem to be strongly favoured over governments in this respect.

The second principle is that local-level NGOs in the South are the main sources of countervailing power to that of the state, and are to be supported as such. They form the 'part of society which links individuals to the public domain and to the state – meaning the political dimension of society'. They

> allow people to participate in economic and social activities, and organize themselves in powerful groups able to influence public policies and to access public resources, in particular in favour of the poor. They can constitute a countervailing power to that of government.
>
> (UNDP 1997c)

The international agencies that are given the task of helping NGO networks in the South exercise this role as a countervailing power, by such means as ensuring a favourable legislative environment and adequate financing.

As we have seen, at IDO's New York headquarters in 1994, actors in the regional office were still in the process of developing norms and standards: they had to invent programming for a Second World which until then had not been among the beneficiaries of development aid. At the time, the IDO actors observed in this study were unclear about how to 'democratize' and 'develop' the former USSR, even less about the notion of good governance as it was presented to them, but aware that they were being asked to put it into practice. As we will see, this conundrum provides the core of our story: how these actors 'invented' the practices that made the notion real.

Good governance and HIV

At the New York office, requests for aid from countries of central Asia and the Caucasus cause many a discussion and often spark difficult debates, some of them noisy or confused. They also give rise to proposals for action, all of them thought to be essential, on themes ranging from the environment in post-Chernobyl Ukraine to the reform of Armenia's education system. Despite the confusion, a theme emerges as the agencies' local antennae in central Asia and the Caucasus transmit the needs expressed by governments to the New York office. Their requests converge around assistance to fight the HIV/AIDS epidemic. At this stage of negotiation, nothing else is specified. The requests cause a number of debates, lasting several months. They take place among small groups in countries around the world. People talk during conferences and in workshops, but also away from these formal venues of reflection, 'behind the scenes' and in corridors, by electronic mail or in internal documents. Participating in these debates, I quickly remark that they occur in fits and starts, for example with the appearance of a question-and-answer document providing guidance on whether a given HIV-related activity in the ex-USSR would be legitimate, and if so, in what form to provide it.

Even before IDO starts to work in ex-Soviet countries, team members need, de facto, to have at hand a body of collective analysis, shared visions that can clarify and support their future activities. The results of this preparatory stage – the evolution of which we will follow through their discovery of local realities, their comportment and their choices – are not reduced to the simple sum of their reflections and exchanges. They arise from a particular environment, that of the institution they represent. Their discourse and professional practices are based in this specific institutional culture.

Looking for precedents

To find the bases for decision-making through consensus, agency staff members in charge of programmes in the ex-USSR examine internal documents providing the general institutional directives which guide its actions in the rest of the world.[10] They find there the first building blocks needed for the ideological construction of their future activities.

The debates among the New York team hinge on two major points. The first: is HIV/AIDS a development problem? The second: if HIV/AIDS is a development problem, what are the current 'best practices' (to use agency vocabulary) available around the world for HIV prevention, particularly in low-prevalence epidemics such as that of the former USSR? In response to these two questions, members of the New York team begin to pave the way for what will become, over the years, enshrined in institutional ideology.

The first discussion is about which approach to the problem should be taken: does HIV/AIDS fit exclusively within the field of health, being a medical concern? If so, why should the agency get involved with prevention, since its mandate is development and not health, which is the preserve of another big international development agency? A form of political correctness dominates this first stage of debate. Opinions are divided. Some actors at New York headquarters consider the HIV/AIDS epidemic a problem of disease and treatment, and therefore not a direct fit with the agency's mandate. For others, it is an appropriate theme for development activities, and agencies not specializing in health may also legitimately get involved. Consensus is quickly found by referring to internal guidelines. These confirm the second group's opinion: that HIV is not purely a concern for the health sector; it is also 'a development problem', because the impact of this epidemic in developing countries must be understood 'in the context of crucial social and economic problems already facing these countries' inhabitants. Not only should this phenomenon be tackled directly by development programmes, but its consequences will have a bearing on all the existing development initiatives, which will need to be rethought.'

Following this logic, HIV/AIDS is a matter of sustainable development, and not just health, and the agency is therefore able to entertain requests for assistance from governments.

With efficiency in mind, the team then turns its attention to avoiding needlessly reproducing any activities being carried out in the ex-USSR by other international development agencies. In the process of becoming informed about these possible programmes, IDO representatives quickly realize that in the countries concerned, relevant agency activities are limited, with small budgets and few staff. Above all, they find that such activities are mostly limited to heightening awareness among a few local managers within the Ministry of Health, using a highly medicalized approach to prevention of sexually transmitted infections (STIs) and HIV.

The New York actors then ask themselves which HIV prevention practices are considered the best in the world. Clearly, they cannot blindly replicate the HIV prevention activities carried out by IDO in other developing countries. This debate is central in 1994–95, when the former Soviet Republics have only just fallen into the category of developing countries. As we have seen, the agency's involvement there is very recent, and in the field of HIV, as in all the others, everything must yet be defined: the way the agency will conduct its work, its choice of projects, its methods of assistance and so on. An international review of HIV prevention programmes undertaken by the New York team, focusing on low-level epidemics (such as that in the ex-USSR in 1994–95), revealed a peculiar phenomenon: the major involvement of NGOs.

NGOs in the fight against AIDS

From the beginning of the HIV epidemic, NGOs were quick to respond to this unknown virus. Its particular characteristics, its transmission through intimate (and sometimes taboo) behaviour, quickly prompted both health professionals and those infected with the virus to agree that little of value could be expected from conventional health policies (Altman 1994). Public health systems and government agencies showed themselves ill-suited to reaching stigmatized and marginalized population groups (often clandestine ones), and getting them to change long-established habits, or to mobilize voluntary collective action, particularly during the first years of the epidemic. Shortly after the first press articles appeared in 1981 describing a new illness suffered by young male homosexuals in the United States, many gay men began to organize themselves. GMHC (Gay Men's Health Crisis) in New York was one of the first of a long list of NGOs created worldwide, not only in North America, Europe and Australia but also in developing countries such as Mexico, Zambia and Thailand. Many of the first American activists were not infected, or did not know their serological status when they joined. These movements were founded on solidarity and mutual support.

In the United States in particular, where the Reagan administration was widely accused of ignoring AIDS during the crucial few years after the epidemic first appeared, NGOs emphasized the importance of political representation and advocacy on behalf of homosexuals. The American model – which owed a lot to the gay heritage of 'coming out of the closet' – strongly influenced the global development of NGOs in the fight against HIV/AIDS.[11] American homosexuals were the first to bring together and disseminate credible HIV prevention messages to their peers. One of the 'founding documents' of the response – the 1983 declaration drafted by a group of 'People with AIDS' during a national forum on AIDS in Denver – emphasized the importance of engaging HIV-positive people using the language of feminist struggle and gay liberation, as well as the precepts of 'patient empowerment'.[12] The Denver Principles strongly promoted the use of the term 'people with AIDS' rather than 'victims' or 'sick people' (the generally accepted term is now 'people living with HIV/AIDS' (PLWHA)). They also emphasized the need for real representation of those directly concerned, at all levels of policy, in the fight against the epidemic (Altman 1994).

With the growing number of infections registered in central and western Africa, groups of HIV-positive people came together in NGOs such as TASO (The AIDS Service Organization) in Uganda, and in Western and non-Western NGOs, establishing tight international cooperation in the search for responses to the epidemic. In Africa the first responses often consisted of helping families with sick or dying young adults, who received only very inadequate medical services.[13] Whatever its value on an analytical level, the distinction between specialized and non-specialized NGOs in the prevention of HIV is, in reality, often rather blurred. In a large number of cases, the fight against HIV has given rise to NGOs among groups that had never been formally organized in associations, such as drug users or prostitutes. These NGOs were able to develop activities covering most aspects of the disease: treatment and palliative care, prevention awareness, education, help with daily living, lobbying health sector managers in defence of patients' interests, and in the domains of social security, scientific research and employment. Prevention activities – creating messages for target groups such as youth, homosexuals, prostitutes or the general public – were taken on by such groups at a very early stage. The varied methods used showed a real capacity for invention and creation: posters and leaflets, open meetings in the workplace, care, leisure activities and even street theatre or outreach in bars. For example, in 1987 a Thai dancer and some friends formed a dance troupe which brought together traditional dance and theatre to take prevention awareness to the staff and clients in bars of Bangkok. This was reproduced both in Thailand and elsewhere in the world. The same artist then created a drop-in centre and took prevention activities to the parks, saunas and other places where homosexuals met. Another local group adapted this approach for work with prostitutes. Similar activities began in Australia, Mexico, Netherlands and the United States.[14]

The priority for the first NGOs active in the fight against the epidemic was helping the sick. This gave rise to numerous other home-based help and support activities (as opposed to hospitalization) during a period when the care provided by health institutions was still inadequate, particularly in protecting the 'quality of life' of those in the terminal phases of AIDS.[15] In the United States, the key role of the 'buddy' was born: a volunteer capable of treating a stranger as a friend, who actively helped the sick person in his or her daily life (Dan Bailey, cited in Katoff and Ince 1991: 552). This voluntary work could consist of doing all the shopping for the patient's everyday life, but also of listening to 'their anxiety and suffering' (Dan Bailey, cited by Altman 1994). The advent of the AIDS buddy – the archetypal voluntary worker – also changed the way home care was provided by institutions through nurses, housekeepers and social workers. The buddy is the patient's de facto advocate with these professionals, the 'expert' regarding the needs of the sick individual with the same status as the other experts (e.g., the physiotherapist, the doctor or the social worker). The buddy often serves as the patient's intermediary, demanding that the professionals adapt *their* practices, making the patient's needs, comfort and quality of life the centre of attention rather than the usual exigencies of working in a team. Although today's health institutions commonly practice 'patient-centred' care and treatment, historically this is a direct result of the fact that many professionals were – unwillingly to begin with – challenged by AIDS patients or by their *buddies* as they articulated their needs and feelings and defended their interests.

Set up by the patients themselves, by those close to them or by common citizens not personally affected by the disease, AIDS support groups soon set up advocacy strategies aimed at putting pressure on government health policies, fighting against discrimination, fundraising or raising public opinion (Altman 1994: 53). This movement rose in reaction to the many forms of discrimination that people living with HIV/AIDS faced in the early years of the epidemic: HIV-positive children refused admission to nursery or primary schools; young people refused a job because the pre-employment medical examination showed that they were HIV-positive or because they had – as was their legal right – refused to be examined; workers dismissed with the threat of making their HIV-positive condition public knowledge; people refused treatment by health institutions. Access to treatment also became an important area for NGOs, as advances in treatment introduced a new element in the struggle, one crucial to the redefinition of the HIV/AIDS phenomenon: although the epidemic touches all countries, access to treatment varies widely depending on the state of the health systems in different countries. The movement ACT UP (AIDS Coalition to Unleash Power) exemplifies a radical approach to putting pressure on the pharmaceutical industry. ACT UP was founded in 1987 in New York by activists convinced that treatment research was under-funded and held up by bureaucratic red tape. This group, with its often spectacular media-grabbing activities, was rapidly reproduced in Europe and elsewhere. The impact of this activist movement was considerable and, through dynamic and carefully targeted pressure on pharmaceutical companies and state agencies responsible for authorizing the introduction of new medications, had a strong influence on the long-term access of patients to new treatments.

Though the vast scale of NGO activity in prevention support for infected and affected persons is universally recognized, the phenomenon is difficult to quantify, and the exact number of all the NGOs engaged in the fight against HIV/AIDS is not known. In 1992, approximately six thousand were counted in the United States alone. Using a broad definition of the term NGO, there were about two hundred in Africa and five hundred in Latin America in the same period (Mann *et al.* 1995: 187).

Apart from their number, the most notable fact about this movement was the remarkable similarity between NGOs from one country to another. Many observers noticed the international dimension of the phenomenon:[16]

> No other illness has enlisted such a variety of skills and communities to organize against it. In countries ranging from Kenya to Thailand to the Dominican Republic, sex workers have developed programs to educate and support fellow prostitutes and their clients. In the tolerant cities of Switzerland and the Netherlands, but also in the urban ghettos of Newark and Camden in the USA, communities have sought to restrict infection amongst needle users, whilst in India and Argentina, against horrendous obstruction and persecution, people with the virus themselves have struggled to organize against discrimination and ignorance.
> (Altman 1994: 3)

Thus, HIV/AIDS brought with it an unprecedented mobilization of NGOs around the world. While the main part of their work had two central foci (prevention of the epidemic and support for those it affects), the work was not limited to providing services. They also undertook ongoing discussions with governments and health providers. It was through this interaction that the majority of actors got to know each other, particularly as a result of two interrelated types of experience. The first was their confrontation with a strong conservative opposition that rejected any legitimation of homosexuality, prostitution, drug use, needle exchanges and so on, or even the recognition of HIV-positive persons as legitimate actors in the fight against the epidemic. The second was their challenge to the protective barriers surrounding professional, medical and governmental status. This occurred as HIV-positive persons presented themselves, via their NGOs, as active protagonists rather than passive objects of medical practice or state health policies. Their ability to organize themselves independently helped to move HIV/AIDS out of the purely medical domain and to redefine it in terms of sexual emancipation, the fight against prejudice and social exclusion, lifestyle choices, equality of the sexes, human rights and citizenship. These two types of experience increasingly resulted in the recognition and empowerment of marginalized populations such as prostitutes, homosexuals, drug users and, more generally, women, children and the poor (Aggleton *et al.* 1997, 1999).

As Altman clearly shows, empowerment of persons affected by the virus has shaken certain dominant discourses on society, which had previously given a monopoly of power to scientific and medical authorities. For this reason, the majority of NGOs working on the worldwide response to HIV/AIDS think of themselves as being fundamentally subversive in relation to the state (Altman 1994).

In this context, it is understandable that IDO's New York actors came to consider HIV/AIDS-related NGOs as the holy grail for development workers. As seen earlier, the idea that communities should participate in their own development was fundamental to their work, at least in theory. All the New York team members accepted this approach, and at a conceptual level the activities developed by NGOs in the global response to HIV/AIDS seemed to fit perfectly with IDO's objectives. Especially since supporting local NGOs – assumed to be a countervailing power to that of the state – offered the additional advantage of promoting, by their example, good governance in the ex-USSR. And who could argue with the idea of saving innocent lives?

2 The legacy

After much debate, the first stage in building IDO's institutional ideology is concluded in New York with the decision to support local NGOs in anti-HIV/AIDS work and, in so doing, help establish good governance in Central Asia and the Caucasus. Armed with this overall guideline, IDO members begin the second stage of developing their institutional ideology. As they systematically meet the actors engaged in fighting the epidemic, they discover a very specific context in the region, which is linked, among other factors, to the legacy of the Soviet era: only state institutions are currently active in HIV prevention work. Moreover, government officials remain convinced adherents of the strategies used in the Soviet response to the epidemic (and before it, to controlling sexually transmitted infections) – strategies which were also mechanisms of social control.

Eldar is the state secretary for AIDS in one country of the region. He is in his early 40s. His suit jackets, several sizes too large, could accommodate rows of medals. For some reason, he tends to keep his overcoat and fur hat on even while sitting at his desk. On his vast desk sit three telephones, each a different colour, the use of which he insists on explaining to his visitors: an internal line, an external line and a direct line to the Minister himself. Behind him a large glass bookcase displays Soviet medical and scientific publications, carefully arranged by size.

Today he has brought together the heads of the Ministry teams directly involved in HIV control. The meeting has two objectives: to show the existence and the strength of the national model for containing the epidemic, and to make clear to the development agency that such a well-organized campaign merits strong financial support.

All present are medically qualified Ministry of Health officials; according to the Soviet model, only medical and paramedical professionals are equipped to deal with HIV/AIDS. Never mind that the vast majority of them have never met an HIV-positive person, primarily due to the virus' extremely low prevalence in the country, a fact of which the state secretary is proud. He states categorically that there is no HIV infection in his country, and this is proof that the government's chosen strategy is the right one:

QED. Clearly he is nostalgic about the Soviet past, and in particular the HIV control system, which is still theoretically in place but without funding.

ELDAR: 'Today mass compulsory testing is no longer undertaken ... Of course our doctors still try to fight AIDS and to track down infected persons, but it is no longer systematic. We no longer have the means.'

ONE OF ELDAR'S DEPUTIES (*attempting to stop this train of thought, which he knows not to be in line with international guidelines*): 'That is what we were doing in the past. Now everything is anonymous and voluntary!'

Members of the IDO ask about the methodologies used in this voluntary testing. It turns out that in reality, anonymity is barely respected and that the state's medical personnel systematically try to learn the names of sexual partners of persons diagnosed with HIV.

ONE OF ELDAR'S COLLEAGUES: 'It is better for everybody that seropositive persons inform us about their sexual partners. At the very least, it is preferable to letting them continue to infect whomever they want, don't you think? These people are examined and questioned for their own good, as well as for that of society. We contact their family members and their sexual partners. With the help of the police, of course.'

ELDAR: 'As you see, our approach on prevention is very clear, emphasizing the importance of anonymous and voluntary testing.'

ANNA: 'But it is neither voluntary nor anonymous ...'

ELDAR (*interrupting her*): 'Our goal is to avert the epidemic. This means controlling dangerous populations: homosexuals, foreigners, drug users, prostitutes, seropositive people ...'

ONE OF HIS COLLEAGUES (*describing the case of a prostitute who is arrested and brought to a health centre for an obligatory HIV test, which turns out to be positive*): 'She had a notebook with the names of her clients. We called them all.'

ANNA: 'Did she hand over the notebook voluntarily?'

ELDAR (*annoyed*): 'Yes, voluntarily! I did not force her to do it! And when the police called the clients, 70 per cent came in for testing. That is patriotism!'

ONE OF HIS COLLEAGUES: 'Perhaps you could help us to reconstruct the Soviet system of HIV control? That is the only efficient way of fighting the virus ... We would need equipment to reinstate mass testing and to isolate dangerous cases, and of course money to pay the salaries of state health employees. Since Soviet republics became independent, everything has fallen apart.'

ANOTHER COLLEAGUE: 'And we must re-establish links between the police in the various republics. In the old days, the same police system was in place throughout the whole of the Soviet territory. That meant we could do effective contact tracing.'

ELDAR: 'If an infected person was detected here, and that person had stayed in Uzbekistan, or even Ukraine, we contacted the Uzbek or Ukrainian police forces and they worked with ours to find close family and friends of the detected case. But today, because of independence, all of that is gone! Our police forces no longer work together, and if we have a case here, we can only search for the partners and friends in our country, not beyond the republic's frontiers. This is very bad for controlling the epidemic! We need your money to revive the Soviet system of fighting AIDS. If you give it to us, we guarantee you zero per cent AIDS in the region!'

The Caucasus and Central Asia

IDO's decision to treat the republics of the southern USSR as a single region brings together the Central Asian countries of Kazakhstan, Kyrgyzstan, Tajikistan, Turkmenistan and Uzbekistan, and the three countries of the Caucasus – Azerbaijan, Armenia and Georgia.[1] The latter three are part of the most unstable area of the ex-USSR. The Caucasus has became the symbol of disorder with its wars, political irregularities, armed clashes between political adversaries, widespread terrorism, lack of security in large towns and transportation routes, and 'loss of state control in some provinces which move increasingly towards autarchy' (Urjewwick 1993: 253; Schoeberlein 2000b).

This immense region, which had been tied to Russia by the force of arms and colonial economic pressure, underwent an 'historic upheaval' with the fall of the USSR (Poujol 1992, 1993, 2004). The chaotic conditions of early independence following 1991 had their roots in the very conditions in which these republics were created and managed by central authority. Unlike Eastern European countries, which had enjoyed a period of sovereignty and real national existence before Soviet domination, the 'making of nations' (Roy 1997) in Central Asia and the Caucasus was slow, laborious and full of conflict. Indeed, these new states had to 'invent' a national identity from a tapestry of Russian colonial and Soviet history.

In a continuation of tsarist policies, the USSR 'territorialized' nations, both large and small, into a system of federal republics, administrative territories and regions (*oblast*), for the most part following arbitrary criteria (Schoeberlein 2000a). The merit of this patchwork was its manageability by one centralized power, withholding any independent authority from national-territorial governments and parliaments. The Soviet federal structure was therefore conceived as an administrative *matryoshka* doll which supported centralization of the state (Mendras 1992). The policy of nationalities served above all to break up existing allegiances.

> For that reason a multitude of 'minor peoples' was created. The aim was clearly not to make these new peoples into viable nation-states; on

> the contrary, it was to reduce them and all the other peoples to purely administrative facades, and thereby prepare their fusion into the grand Soviet whole.
>
> (Roy 1997: 9)

This arbitrary structure was justified by Soviet authorities' certainty that the whole empire was sacred and unshakeable, and a precursor to universal sovietization. The interior borders from then on had a purely administrative character. The 'internationalizing fraternity of the Soviet peoples', a paradigm of the future world communist system, prevented borders from engendering national unrest (Strada 1992). In addition, the cultural, ethnic, linguistic and religious diversity of the peoples making up the new Soviet Union was partially smothered by the drive towards uniformity of *Homo sovieticus*. As one observer put it, 'the similarities of socialist institutions imposed a layer of uniformity on top of all this diversity' (Hann 2002b: 8). This administrative framework was backed by the weight of Russian as a common language at all levels, within the army, the education system and employment policy.

This common framework also served as a system of social protection that ensured social assistance to the needy and social insurance in the form of a pension for all. For example, in rural Uzbekistan,

> membership of rural enterprises (*sovkhozy* – state farms, and *kolkhozy* – collective farms) comprised entitlements to household plots, housing, welfare benefits (pension, maternity and disability benefits) and access to kindergartens. Consumer Cooperative Associations provided access to subsidized essential foodstuffs, marketing outlets for surplus private production, vocational training and services, Trade Unions provided pension and sickness benefits, access to household durables and free holidays. Organs of the Communist party such as the Women's Committee and the Youth Committee played an adjunct role by protecting members' interests and providing vocational training.
>
> (Kandiyoti 2004: iii)

With such a legacy, the shock of independence was a brutal one. Neither the governments nor the peoples of Central Asia actually chose to leave the Second World. In fact, when governments in the region held referendums earlier in 1991 asking their populations whether they wanted to stay part of the USSR, the response was 'overwhelmingly positive' (Schoeberlein 2000c: 57). But faced with a fait accompli, each population had to create new 'social contracts' within their territories (Ferro 1993; Motyl 1992a, b and c, 1995; Sapir 1993a, b and c). For example, Kyrgyzstan had to invent a 'national identity' which had never before existed. Using criteria based on ethnicity was inconceivable without risking civil war, as the country comprised twenty-nine ethnic groups (many of which had been deported there by Stalin). The inhabitants registered as being of Kyrgyz 'origin' (a term to consider with caution) only represent 64.9 per cent of the population. Russians and Uzbeks account for approximately 13 per cent each, and the country also contains substantial numbers of ethnic Germans, Ukrainians, Koreans, Tajiks, Dungan and Uyghurs.[2] All were Soviet citizens until the beginning of the 1990s, when they suddenly found themselves to be Kyrgyz. Products of Russian and then Soviet colonial history, the newly independent states now urgently needed to create an identifiable nationality in an explosive political, economic and social context (Luong-Jones 2002, 2004; Poujol 1993; Schoeberlein 2002).

The current shape of political power in the region is best understood in light of this recent past (Geiss 2006; Laruelle and Peyrouse 2006; Peyrouse 2004; Tolipov 2006). In Turkmenistan, that country of extremes, the Communist Party agreed to disband at its last meeting on the morning of 16 December 1991. They then broke for lunch, and returned and established the People's Democratic Party of Turkmenistan. As Gleason notes, 'within months the Democratic Party had a membership of nearly 52,000, of whom 48,000 were former communists' (Gleason 1998: 116). In the mid-1990s when my research began, many of the old chieftains of the communist system had on the whole retained power in the independent republics. Most of the heads of state were national first secretaries of the Communist Party before 1991, and became presidents either by vote of the old regime's parliaments, in single candidate elections or through a truly 'Soviet' performance like Saparmurat Niyazov in Turkmenistan, who won 99.5 per cent of votes in 1992 (Mandrillon 1993). The next decade saw strong personalization of presidential power, even if this power was supposedly balanced by counter-powers such as parliaments and constitutional courts (Poujol 2004). President Niyazov organized a referendum in 1994 which allowed him to remain in power for five more years, then arranged in 1999 to be elected as Turkmenistan's 'President for Life' through 'consultation of the people' (*Khal Maslahaty*). The same strategy was used by the Kazakh President Nursultan Nazarbayev in 1995, the Tajik president Emomali Rakhmonov in 1999 and 2003, the Uzbek president Islom Karimov in 1995 and 2002, and the Kyrgyz president Askar Akayev in 1996 and 2003. In Azerbaijan, President Heydar Aliyev, who had held power in the country for decades as First Secretary of the Communist Party and then as the independent republic's president, appointed his son Ilham to the presidency in 2003. Meanwhile in most parts of the region, the press is kept under surveillance and members of the opposition are imprisoned, in exile, or marginalized or consistently gagged through registration procedures: various ministries regularly ask parties to present a number of documents to ascertain their legality, to which unclear or unfixed criteria are applied and which can be used to suddenly declare their parties illegal and to imprison their leaders (Laruelle and Peyrouse 2006).

Aside from politics, the end of the Soviet system had important consequences for the health and quality of life of populations (Sievers 2003). The former social welfare system had provided everyone with the security of full employment, price controls on basic goods and free access to education and healthcare.[3] The USSR had established a large number of industries in certain towns or regions, which had not only provided employment but also health and social services and social security. Suddenly, subsidies from Moscow were cut and 'virtually all enterprises that had previously been supplied by, or produced outputs to, the Soviet economic ministerial network were closed down' (Schoeberlein 2000c: 57). Industrial production fell faster than the already substantial drop in gross domestic product (GDP).[4] The fall in social security spending was catastrophic when combined with the collapse in GDP, as it meant that real spending on social protection declined precipitately. Governments were unable to maintain even minimal levels of public services and social welfare protection, never mind the many benefits to which citizens had been accustomed before independence. As public education, health care and pension systems fell apart, 'a relatively egalitarian social structure [was] destroyed' (Rasizade 2002: 357).[5] All those who depended directly on the state budget – the retired, disabled, unemployed, government employees, the military – experienced a sudden fall in their standard of living. Since 1991, poverty among the middle classes and rural populations has grown. In Kyrgyzstan, for example, one person in two lived below the poverty line in 2000, and one in six suffered from malnutrition – and this according to official data, which sometimes bears little resemblance to the reality visible in the country.[6] Across the region, the parallel economy grew as real salaries plummeted (when these were paid at all), giving rise to trafficking of all types. In addition to the rising criminality documented in police statistics, there has been a sharp increase of bribery of all kinds (Rasizade 2002) and a general feeling of insecurity, which in turn is fed by the explosion of tabloid newspapers and sensationalist television programmes (Favarel-Garigues 2003).

The effects on public health were also catastrophic, with real health expenditures diminishing by nearly half (Shkolnikov *et al.* 2001). In 1960 the USSR dedicated 6.6 per cent of its GNP to health expenditure. This fell to 4.6 per cent in 1985 and to 1.7 per cent in 1994 (for all former USSR countries). In 2000, the average for the new republics was around 2 per cent. The budget reductions brought drastically reduced salaries for health personnel – who emigrated en masse – and severe cuts in funding for supplies of materials and medicines (Adeyi *et al.* 1997; Healy and Mckee 1997). The cost of health care increased due to privatization and commercialization of many health care services, and these costs were no longer borne by the state but by households (i.e., from private savings and the labour of family members). Health indicators worsened in all countries of the region, demonstrating the indirect effects of economic decline on public health (Buckley 2002).[7] Dramatic examples include the increase in cases of pneumonia due to heating restrictions, and a very clear rise in tuberculosis, cholera, typhus, meningitis and other infectious diseases formerly under control in the region (Hohman 2004; Hohman and Garenne 2005).

The following observations illustrate this transformation: It is market day in V., a small town in Central Asia. In the town square a crowd gathers, chiefly composed of unemployed men standing in small, compact groups. The muddy square is a testament to lack of funds for repairing the road system. This scene is not uncommon in the region.

In the butcher shop, some enormous pieces of meat are displayed behind the counter. But there are few people in front of it. Meat is expensive.

It is as if a 'modern' industrialized country's entire infrastructure had been neglected for twenty years. The surrounding buildings are dilapidated, evidence of lack of maintenance. Though still solid, they often lack electricity due to long power cuts, decaying equipment or the cables having been torn out to be used elsewhere or sold. Even when the electricity system does function in these working class apartments, there is no gas or hot water. The children play between the apartment blocks or in play areas where slides, swings and so on are also half destroyed.

Elderly men in threadbare suits wander aimlessly or stand around chatting. Some of them wear many medals on their chests, won during the Great Patriotic War of 1941–45. There are also those who try to earn a bit of money by selling whatever they have – clothing, kitchenware, a tool, placed on the ground on a piece of cloth or a plastic bag – to those richer than themselves, or at least less poor.

Nearby stand three women, dignified, with their shawls covering their heads. Some sell the same used objects as their neighbours, while others offer homemade cakes, fresh milk in glass demijohns, or round loaves of bread. Finally, a very old woman, indifferent and embarrassed at the same time, sits behind a child's plastic table displaying pornographic magazines to the passersby. Not the softened, pretentiously artistic images displayed in European magazine shops – no, these are hard, crude, brutal photos, each of them as sad and violent as the other. People glance at her without apparent judgement. Nothing but a vague and silent comprehension, commiseration perhaps, as if each one here knew very well just how far people are capable of going in order to survive.

The HIV/AIDS epidemic

In the early years the HIV epidemic in the former USSR was virtually unnoticed, due in part to the low rates of infection and also because other difficulties held the attention of both the population and their governments (Medvedev 1990; Pokrovskii *et al.* 1990). Between 1988 and 1994, public health officials played down the threat of the virus, referring always to the very low number of people affected. The 1988 wave of HIV infections in children at a hospital in the town of Elista was considered an exceptional event. Even in the mid-1990s many public health experts in the region agreed that infection was 'stable' in their countries. The general tendency was to believe that with the wide range of measures set up in the 1980s, the situation would remain unchanged.

The explosion

No one was taking into account the consequences of the socio-economic transformation that was under way. In the mid-1990s, HIV incidence began to skyrocket, confirming studies which link international poverty and social vulnerability with HIV/AIDS in the region (Atlani 1998, Atlani-Duault 2005b; Atlani *et al.* 2000; Barnett and Whiteside 1997; Barnett, Ivanov and Slay 2004; Barnett *et al.* 2000; Buckley 2005a, 2005b; Danziger 1996; Dehne *et al.* 2000; Field 2004; Godinho *et al.* 2004, 2005; Hamers 1997, 2000; Hamers and Downs 2003; Rhodes *et al.* 1999, World Bank 2005). The region is experiencing the world's fastest-growing HIV/AIDS epidemic (Adeyi 2003). According to recent figures, some 1,600,000 inhabitants of the former USSR and Eastern Europe are living with the virus today, an increase of almost twenty-fold in less than ten years. AIDS claimed almost twice as many lives in 2005 compared to 2003, and killed an estimated 62,000 adults and children (Barnett *et al.* 2004; UNAIDS 2004b). According to the 2008 UNAIDS global report on the epidemic, only sub-Saharan Africa and the Caribbean had higher prevalence rates at the end of 2005 (UNAIDS 2006).

In Central Asia and the Caucasus region, more specifically, more than 80 per cent of HIV-positive persons in the region are 30 or younger, strongly contrasting with a figure of approximately 30 per cent in Western Europe and the United States. In Kazakhstan and Kyrgyzstan, 70 per cent of persons diagnosed with HIV are less than 20 years of age (UNAIDS 2003). The epidemic also strikes hardest at those who are most socially vulnerable: in Kazakhstan, for example, three-quarters of HIV-positive persons are unemployed.

The countries most affected by the epidemic are Kazakhstan and Uzbekistan. According to recent statistics from UNODC (2005a), in December 2005 Uzbekistan had 7,757 recorded cases of HIV infection and Kazakhstan had 5,440 cases. For the moment, the epidemic is less serious in Kyrgyzstan and Tajikistan. In Kyrgyzstan, 807 cases of HIV infection had been officially reported in December 2005, while in Tajikistan the figure was 506 cases. Nevertheless, care must be taken when citing official statistics, as real infection rates are probably higher than those declared. International estimates such as those produced in 2002 by the United States Centers for Disease Control estimate that these figures should be multiplied by at least ten to approach the true rate of infection.

Perhaps more important than the absolute numbers of infected persons is the explosive increase in HIV incidence (new infections) in Central Asia and the Caucasus. For example, Kazakh official statistics show a 238 per cent rise in the rate of infection between 2000 and 2001 (CDC/CAR 2002). These figures should be taken with caution, as the real rates of infection are almost certainly higher (Barnett and Whiteside 2002). There are a number of reasons for questioning official data. According to the regulations still in use (even if they are no longer official doctrine) in countries of the former USSR, an HIV-positive case is only officially recorded if the individual undergoes two blood tests and a clinical examination. A large number of cases almost certainly go unrecorded, either because these procedures are not followed, or because health services do not have the necessary logistical resources to carry them out, or do not publish reliable reports. Other problems are pointed out by observers such as Hamers (1997, 2000, 2003), who comments that in Ukraine, for example, '[s]ince IDUs tested are those officially registered as such by the police, they probably represent a biased sample of all IDUs' (Hamers 1997). This is equally applicable to other countries of the ex-USSR, Central Asia and the Caucasus included.

The HIV epidemic is so far less severe in Kyrgyzstan and Tajikistan. In both countries, over half of all HIV diagnoses to date were recorded in 2004. This is mostly explained by increased testing (EuroHIV, 2005). Turkmenistan is a special case, as it is impossible to find reliable data on the prevalence of HIV within its borders. Since May 2004 it has been prohibited to publicly discuss certain diseases such as tuberculosis, dysentery, cholera or hepatitis (Anonymous, in the *Lancet* 2003; Rechel and McKee 2005). In the Caucasus, the epidemics are relatively stable in Armenia and Azerbaijan, although sudden increases in HIV transmission remain possible. At the end of 2003, the levels of reported AIDS cases per 100,000 were 0.26 in Armenia, 0.24 in Azerbaijan and 0.83 in Georgia (Buckley 2005b). Officially, the number of people living with HIV in the Caucasus is 1,200, but Buckley (2005b) estimates the total number between 3,500 and 19,100 at the end of 2003.

Determinants of the epidemic

To forecast the directions of HIV spread in Central Asia and the Caucasus, more needs to be known about the dynamics of the HIV/STD epidemic, the sexual mixing patterns, and so on. Fundamental data and cross-disciplinary studies in the region are lacking that might establish the link between social dimensions of risky behaviour and specific aspects of the drastic changes in organizational, institutional, health and economic conditions in the former USSR. In addition, this supposes a shift from a narrow epidemiological perspective – still favoured by many – to a much broader comprehensive approach that should include more qualitative and quantitative work on behaviours and vulnerability factors. Individual behaviours occur in complex socio-economic and cultural contexts, and analysis that removes them from their broader settings ignores essential influences (Kendall 1991, 1995).

With the collapse of the Soviet Union, it is virtually impossible to disengage individual risk behaviour from environmental and economic factors in determining and understanding vulnerability to HIV. In this chapter, we discuss selected aspects of the determinants and dynamics of the new HIV epidemic in Central Asia and the Caucasus, where the societal changes were deepest and most sudden.

The principal driver of the spread of HIV in the region is injecting drug use. But in some countries sexual transmission is more and more common, particularly among drug users and their partners.[8]

The lure of drug use

Injecting drug use is a highly efficient mode of transmission of the virus. This, more than any other factor, explains why the epidemic is currently spreading at such high rates among injecting drug users in the region.

In 2001–2, some 70 per cent of cases of infection were found among intravenous drug users, compared to 28 per cent for the period 1987–95, when sexual transmission was predominant (WHO 2003). In 2004, according to official statistics, 84 per cent of new HIV infections in Kazakhstan were due to injecting drug use, 82 per cent in Uzbekistan, and 86 per cent in Tajikistan. Data published in May 2005 suggest this is also the case for 80 per cent of new infections in Kyrgyzstan (UNAIDS 2006). In Kyrgyzstan, astonishingly, various experts 'estimate that about three of every four IDUs are already HIV-positive' (Godinho *et al.* 2004: 51).

Although the dynamics of transmission among injecting drug users in the region are not fully understood, two of the determining factors are clear: the increase in supply and demand for drugs, and changing methods of consumption.

Over one decade, world production of heroin quadrupled, creating new markets both in producing countries and in places which were once merely transit routes. Such is the case in the former USSR where heroin and the other products derived from the opium poppy (opiates) are much more accessible than before, including from opium poppy cultivated locally. Poppy cultivation and its transformation into opium are escalating in the countries of Central Asia, which are situated on the drug route from Afghanistan, the world's leading supplier. The advent of market economies, new convertible currencies and the opening of borders have made the narcotics trade infinitely easier, transforming drug trafficking into a very lucrative activity for some dealers in the region. Thanks to weakened and corrupt legal structures, organized crime has firmly established itself in the former Soviet countries, and has invested heavily in the production and trafficking (Grund 1996). My own informants paint a picture of regional mafias specialized in narcotics, who work in close liaison with the cartels of the Golden Crescent and Golden Triangle. Brill Olcott and Udalova (2000) highlight the close links between arms trafficking and drugs in the region, and state that more than 90 per cent of heroin sold in Europe is produced in Afghanistan and travels via Central Asia. Moreover, since the downfall of the Taliban in 2001, opium production in Afghanistan has skyrocketed. Some 3,600 tons were produced there in 2002, representing 77 per cent of world production (Chouvy 2002).

This new 'Silk Road' is currently very widely used in the transport of drugs to Europe, the Nordic and Baltic countries, Russia and Ukraine. Based on extrapolations from quantities of drugs seized crossing the Afghan border, around 20 per cent of Afghan opiates – heroin in particular – are sent to Europe via Central Asia and the Caucasus (Chouvy 2006; Goodhand 2000; UNODC Regional Office for Central Asia 2003b). This represents a sizeable amount, given Afghanistan's position as the largest opium producer in the world, with 87 per cent of the world's production in 2005 (UNODC 2005b).

Tajikistan is often the first stopover for Afghan drugs travelling along the Silk Road. The amount of heroin seized by the Tajik authorities is a good indicator of how important this first port of call is: in 2005 alone, nearly four tonnes of heroin were seized (Fenopetov 2006; UNODC Regional Office for Central Asia 2004). Turkmenistan is another country frequently used by drug traffickers (UNODC 2002, UNODC Regional Office for Central Asia 2003a, 2003b). Drugs are transported by land, by sea (the Caspian Sea) or by aeroplanes destined for Azerbaijan and Turkey. Uzbekistan is also an important transit country for Afghan opiates that have already passed through Kyrgyzstan and Tajikistan on their way to Europe (Cornell and Swanström 2006; Townsend 2006).

At the present time, the sale of Afghan drugs in Central Asia represents a market estimated at $30 million (Cornell 2006; Jackson 2005; Makarenko 2002;). This is a minimal sum compared to the profits made from the 're-sale' of drugs passing through Central Asia bound for Russia and other European countries, which are estimated to be $2.2 billion (Fenopetov 2006). However, this market is fast expanding as drug use in Central Asia increases.

At the time of writing, no systematic evaluation has been made of the spread and the determinants of intravenous drug use in Central Asia and the Caucasus. It is known however that the use of narcotics is not a new phenomenon. Opium poppies were cultivated in the former Soviet Union for a long time, and domestic producers are probably the principal sources of opium alkaloids used in the region, particularly Russian or Ukrainian *chornie* (black), *khimiya* (chemical) or *hanka* (opium tar) from Russia or Kazakhstan. The region also produces amphetamine-like substances such as *vint* or *belie*, obtained from ephedra or ephedrine (Rhodes *et al.* 1999). However, in recent years, the situation has changed: heroin has become much more accessible and has overtaken the traditional *hanka*. This shift in the drug of choice is a cause for concern. It seems to have taken place between 2000 and 2001. At the beginning of the year 2000, 70–80 per cent of Kyrgyz injecting drug users who frequented a local organization set up to help drug addicts in Bishkek used opium. By December of the same year, 73 per cent had shifted to heroin and only 26 per cent still used opium. Several factors seem to have provoked this transition. Unlike opium, a product subject to periodic supply shortages, heroin is inexpensive and widely available. Heroin is also thought to have a more powerful effect.

In Kazakhstan alone, the UNODC (2005b) estimates that around 3 per cent of the population, or about 450,000 people, are injecting drug users. This proportion is estimated at 2 per cent in Kyrgyzstan. In Armenia, a country not yet facing an explosive outbreak of cases (as opposed to Kazakhstan), two-thirds of new cases in 2004 were linked to injecting drug use against a backdrop of increasing drug injecting in the country (EuroHIV 2005). As mentioned above, an important feature of drug use in the region is the low age of users. Although few data are available, anecdotal evidence is plentiful. In Kazakhstan, the director of the country's National AIDS Centre recently stated, 'a few years ago nobody could have imagined children eleven years old taking drugs'.[9]

In all post-Soviet countries, young people face a difficult economic environment with little prospect of economic stability. In addition to being discouraged by poverty, the feeling of failure that some experience, in a society that their elders built with such difficulty, causes what is termed the 'trauma of transition' (Atlani *et al.* 2000). It manifests itself in the rejection of whatever is provided by parents or by the institutions inherited from the Soviet era, including information on the dangers of narcotics. At the same time, increased travel and satellite access to Western media offer idealized images of Western youth, whose drug use is more or less explicit. Another manifestation can be seen in 'reactive hedonism' (Grund 1996), in which drugs substitute for, or are added to, existing patterns of alcohol consumption, but without the moderating influences of employment or some degree of hope for a better economic future and a more secure environment. In Kyrgyzstan for example, a dose of heroin costs between 25p and £1, cheaper than a bottle of good vodka.

The sharing of syringes, a high-risk factor in the transmission of HIV, is a widespread practice (Des Jarlais *et al.* 2002).[10] Surveillance studies in Kazakhstan recently found that under half of injecting drug users knew the four main modes of HIV transmission. Just under 60 per cent said they used non-sterile injecting equipment (Kazakhstan AIDS Centre 2005). Other practices facilitate the transmission of the virus, notably methods of drug preparation and distribution. One of the practices widespread among drug users in the region is the 'hire' of injecting equipment in parks and shooting galleries. Another is the purchase of 'ready-made' injections: with age of initiation decreasing to 13 or 14 years of age in some countries, inexperienced users may buy them instead of preparing their own. These are often sold in used or non-sterilized syringes. Drug control professionals call this the 'Odessa syndrome', after the city where it first appeared before spreading to other countries in the region (Atlani *et al.* 2000).

Preparation methods are also risk factors. For both the poppy and opium, users seem to prefer group preparation (two to four people) at home, not only for economizing on product and material but also for solidarity. While waiting to distribute, producers and dealers often keep their preparation in containers which may be contaminated. In addition, users often share prepared doses in small groups with a technique called 'backloading', using one syringe to fill those of the rest of the group (De Jong 1996, 1997). Even if the users have their own syringes, these must be filled by the dealer – often a user too – from his or her syringe or from the original container, increasing the risk of HIV infection (Atlani *et al.* 2000).

A final risk factor is using blood in the preparation of the drug. Many of the users that I have interviewed say that blood acts as an absorbent or neutralizing agent. Others feel that it reduces acidity or serves as a quality test. It may even be added as a stimulant. It is not known exactly how widespread this practice is, but it constitutes an additional risk of HIV infection.

The epidemics are changing shape in parts of the region, with sexually transmitted HIV cases increasingly accounting for new diagnoses. More women are testing positive, often infected by drug-using male partners (UNAIDS 2005). In 2004, unprotected sex accounted for about a third of all newly reported HIV infections (EuroHIV 2005).

Rapid spread of sexually transmitted infections (STIs)

A fresh outbreak of STIs, syphilis in particular, is affecting the whole of the post-Soviet population. This is especially disquieting because STIs can act as a co-factor of HIV infection, and it is feared that it could contribute to a second wave of HIV explosion, after the already significant one occurring among intravenous drug users.

The prevalence of syphilis has risen greatly across the former Soviet territory since the beginning of the 1990s (Atlani *et al.* 2000; Avdeev *et al.* 1994; Barnett, Ivanov and Slay 2004; Barowitz *et al.* 2001; Borisenko *et al.* 1999; Buckley, Barrett and Asminkin 2004; Chervyakov *et al.* 1998; Godinho *et al.* 2005; Hamers and Downs 2003; Kosukhin 1998; Linglof 1995; Renton *et al.* 1998; Shakarishvili and Ryan 2003; Tichonova *et al.* 1997; Westhoff *et al.* 1996). In Kyrgyzstan the official rates of infection multiplied by 77 between 1990 and 1997, and by 140 in the capital Bishkek. In the entire region, levels remain very high. In Central Asia, although rates had fallen by 2003, they remain 10–20 times higher than those observed in Western European countries (Godinho *et al.* 2005). In addition, as Kosukhin (1998) notes and as most local epidemiological authorities recognize, the official figures probably represent only 60 per cent of the real syphilis infection figures, and congenital infections are steadily increasing. Other STIs such as gonorrhoea and chlamydia are also rising. Like HIV, these STI epidemics seem to result from a combination of socio-economic factors, from reduced access to healthcare, and from the legacy of draconian Soviet approaches to contraception and STI treatment. The same factors are behind the drastic increase in tuberculosis cases reported in Central Asia and the Caucasus, mainly in prison populations as in other post-Soviet countries (Farmer 1999).

Sexual taboos

'There is no sex in the Soviet Union' is a catchphrase heard frequently in the region. The phrase refers to a live US–Soviet debate shown on Soviet television in 1988, when a woman gave this response to her American counterpart. Her words became legend among all those who knew the old USSR, and serve to characterize a social and cultural legacy whose consequences on the HIV epidemic are clearly visible.[11]

Indeed, from the beginning of the 1930s, the Communist Party tried to erase all that touched on sexuality, whether in research, education, art or literature (Kon and Riordan 1993: 160). This put an end to a radically different period begun in 1917, when the revolution introduced perhaps the most liberal legislation in Europe, including decriminalization of homosexuality. In 1918 a new marriage code made men and women equal before the law and aimed in the long term to make the family obsolete. In the Stalinist period, however, the family was given a central social role, and was designated by the Party as one of the forces for re-establishing order in everyday life, alongside the police and courts (Goldman 1993). Kon cites George Orwell's *Nineteen Eighty-Four* to underline that this policy for burying sexuality was an integral part of a totalitarian regime:

> It was not merely that the sex instinct created a world of its own that was outside the Party's control and which therefore had to be destroyed if possible. What was more important was that sexual privation induced hysteria, which was desirable because it could be transformed into war-fever and leader-worship ... For how could the fear, the hatred, and the lunatic credulity which the Party needed in its members be kept at the right pitch, except by bottling up some powerful instinct and using it as a driving force? The sex impulse was dangerous to the Party, and the Party had turned it to account.
>
> (Kon 1995: 67)

In their commentary on this aspect of Soviet society Kon and Riordan (1993: 2) wryly observed, 'the population was abandoned to sexual illiteracy, and society became asexual'.

For decades, social conditions and material living standards only amplified the effects of official policy. All cultural expression linked with eroticism was censured, the works of Freud forbidden, and research on sexuality only began again in the 1960s, and remained a marginal area of study. For example, Sergei Golod – who emerged as a leading expert on Russian sexuality after 1991 – undertook a series of sociological studies on the sexual behaviour of adolescents in the late 60s. When he presented his thesis in 1969, the regional committee of the Party in Leningrad and the central committee of Komsomol accused him of 'ideological deviation against Soviet youth', and forced him to rewrite the thesis in its entirety.

Young people received no sexual education in schools, and education officials recommended that parents evade questions asked by their children and re-orient conversations with adolescents towards morality rather than sexuality. Life in communal apartments, where it was not rare for a family comprising parents, children and grandparents to inhabit one single room, did not favour intimacy or sexual relations. In the 1970s, a researcher undertook a study on sex life in the Soviet Union using 140 people who had left the USSR. A large majority of them mentioned lack of individual housing and 'excessive attention' from fellow tenants as serious obstacles (Popovsky 1983). It was nearly impossible for residents of communal apartments to carry on a love affair there. Moreover, on both a legal and practical level, it was impossible to rent a hotel room for two people who were not married, or to stay in a hotel in the city where one lived. Strict limits on internal travel posed another serious obstacle to relations between people, each citizen having a passport and a residency permit obliging them to live in the area designated by the authorities. In summary, finding the time and place for intimacy was a real conundrum for most couples, married or otherwise. For many young people, and for the not-so-young, the only options were to meet in the public parks, cars or at the cinema.

Obviously, such constraints on the emotional and sexual life of several generations made it difficult to develop prevention activities once HIV arrived on the scene. It was particularly difficult to change behaviours towards 'safer sex' with the use of condoms, as these were little used during Soviet times.

Oral contraceptives for women were tried in the USSR in the 1960s but were soon abandoned due to side effects, unlike Western countries where research brought about improvements to reduce these effects. Instead, Soviet authorities chose to favour abortion – authorized in 1956 – as a method for regulating fertility. At the end of the 1980s, official statistics reported six to seven million abortions per year in the entire Soviet Union. By comparison, in 1985 the number of reported abortions per thousand Soviet women of childbearing age was six to ten times higher than in Western countries. Adding in clandestine abortions and cross-tabulating official data with independent sources cited by international organizations, the annual total was more likely in the vicinity of eleven million.

The Soviet policy of favouring abortion as a method of birth control remains current in Central Asia and the Caucasus, being the approach best known to public health authorities and other professionals. Little by little, recent educational programmes are generating a shift from heavy reliance on abortion to the use of contraceptives (mostly IUDs).[12] While IUDs are available and much appreciated, their high costs (as imported products) prevent the majority of women from having access to them. The use of condoms remains low.

In STI control too, the legacy of the Soviet system weighed heavily. A state system for STI control had been in place since the 1950s, with free diagnostic and treatment services. Mass testing was regularly organized, and people diagnosed with an STI were forcibly hospitalized in specialized units guarded by the police. This system ended in the new republics following the fall of the USSR – not due to changed attitudes among health professionals or managers, but primarily for material and financial reasons such as lack of medicines and inability to pay staff. At the time the IDO team arrived, a person with an STI had three possibilities. First, to do 'as before' – go to a state hospital and submit to the Soviet method of contact tracing, forced hospitalization and so on. Second, in order to avoid stigmatization and sanctions, one could purchase treatment in the 'private' sector. This was often in the same hospital as the previous option but at a cost of one or two hundred pounds paid in cash to the state employed doctors, on the understanding that they would respect patient anonymity. This was unaffordable to the great majority of the population, whose average monthly salary was between £20 and £85, depending on the country. The last option was self-medication, with its attendant risks of forgoing expert attention, treatment failure and other complications, especially if the individual is also HIV-positive.

To illustrate: a meeting is held between IDO team and officials in charge of health, one of whom is Eldar, the state secretary for AIDS, in a hospital for STI treatment. Eldar has requested financial and material aid from IDO, to deal with the rise in STIs and to continue HIV prevention as it had been done in Soviet times. In formalities preceding the debate, the IDO team of Beth and Anna ask for more details.

ONE OF ELDAR'S COLLEAGUES: 'If an STI case is identified, our practice is to test the infected patient's partners. If they refuse to come, the police bring them to hospital . . . But since the end of the USSR it is no longer the same. People go to private doctors for treatment, even though it is illegal!'

ANNA: 'Perhaps they want to be tested anonymously?'

ELDAR: 'Perhaps. But it is contrary to the logic of the control system!'

BETH: 'How is syphilis treated in your hospitals?'

CHIEF OF AN STI TREATMENT UNIT: 'With a penicillin injection every four hours, for a period of three to four weeks.' (*Beth is stunned; this corresponds to about 120 injections, much higher than the treatment recommended by the World Health Organization.*)

ANOTHER PARTICIPANT: 'During this period the sick people must remain in a special section of the hospital reserved for STI patients. We also do contact tracing with the police. Unfortunately, today we no longer have the financial means to undertake contact tracing properly! The police can no longer really look for those people close to the patient, or those identified as having had sexual contact with them. Again, it is a question of funds . . .'

ELDAR: 'We need testing equipment and supplies to continue to perform mass testing, and to isolate dangerous cases. As well as money to pay the salaries of civil servants, doctors and the police!'

Later, the team visits an STI treatment unit. The unit is located on the ground floor of a low building. Bars criss-cross the windows. An armed policeman guards the entrance and stops patients from leaving without the necessary authorization. Most of the patients are lying on beds in communal halls, where they receive their penicillin injections every four hours. During this forced stay they must, under the threat of legal sanctions, reveal names of people close to them and their sexual partners. These people, in turn, must also submit to testing. Meanwhile, the IDO actors continue to assert that trust – and particularly trust in the state – is a precondition for public policy aimed at HIV prevention.[13]

Beth and Anna are appalled but not entirely surprised at this glimpse of the draconian system inherited from Soviet times. They chalk up the practices and Eldar's attitudes to the persistence of rigid, authoritarian tendencies from the previous regime and hope to encourage a more participatory environment through Tatiana's circles.

Bridging populations

Throughout the countries of the former USSR, there is concern about the extent to which prostitutes, and drug users who have unprotected sex with non-users, play the role of 'bridging populations' in HIV infection (Atlani *et al.* 2000; Barnett and Whiteside 1997; Barnett, Ivanov and Slay 2004; Barnett *et al.* 2000; Hamers and Downs 2003). The term is used to designate a social group whose practices and serological status constitute both a driver of and risk factor for HIV transmission to the general population.[14]

The question of bridging populations has been treated most seriously in Ukraine (Barnett and Whiteside 1997; Barnett *et al.* 2000). But in all countries of the region, such research as is available shows low levels of protection among drug users during sexual relations, and raises fears of wider infection (Hamers and Downs 2003). The research also suggests that a certain proportion of drug users (both men and women) enter into prostitution. In the other countries in the region, heroin and prostitution are commonly associated, and there is little use of condoms (ibid.). The police also appear to play an important role in this phenomenon. Indeed, my own research suggests that certain police practices and the criminalization of drug use indirectly push users into prostitution. As an arrest for drug use results in a stay in 'treatment' centres (often managed by prison staff from the Ministry of Interior rather than medical professionals), many police officers use this threat to extort money from drug users; in turn, some of the latter resort to prostitution in order to 'finance' the police officers' regular demands for money (Atlani *et al.* 2000).

Although there is very little precise data on sex work in general (Hamers and Downs 2003) and even less on male or adolescent prostitution in Central Asia and the Caucasus, it seems principally driven by the loss of income brought about by the collapse of the Soviet regime. In some cases, however, it is a means of acquiring foreign consumer goods. In Baku, the capital of Azerbaijan, some young girls from wealthy families are secretly prostitutes. Many are students living with their parents, who are unaware of what their daughters are doing. Their motivation is principally financial: prostitution, particularly with foreigners, allows them to buy luxury items. Qualitative research and the high rates of STIs and abortions among these young women indicate that condoms are rarely used (Atlani *et al.* 2000). Nor is this situation limited to Azerbaijan.

Economic crisis has also brought with it seasonal prostitution abroad, in which women and adolescents (and, more rarely, young men) temporarily leave their country to find income elsewhere. This is relatively common in Central Asia and the Caucasus. The principal destinations are Russia, itself currently experiencing a major epidemic of HIV infection, Turkey and Western Europe, where they work for as long as it takes to accumulate a small sum of money, buy merchandise and re-sell it in their countries (some open small businesses on their return). Among those trafficked into prostitution abroad, most of the women coming from the Caucasus are sent to Turkey and the Gulf (Buckley 2005b) while those from Central Asia are mostly sent to the Middle East, the former Soviet states and, increasingly, South and Southeast Asia (Jackson 2005). The sex workers' vulnerability to HIV is high, and made worse by the fact that HIV infection rates in the destination countries are higher than in the countries of origin (Atlani *et al.* 2000). Most are recruited by international prostitution networks, and have little information about the risks involved. Pimps often insist that they submit to whatever their clients want, including not using condoms. For those working independently, the illegal nature of their work exposes them to very hard living conditions and violence; protecting themselves against HIV is not a primary concern (Konings 1996). Although research on condom use in this population is scarce, rates of reported condom use are very low and previous histories of sexually transmitted infection are high (Godinho *et al.* 2004, 2005). Available evidence suggests that among 'call girls' and high-priced prostitutes, as well as those working in massage parlours, hotels, saunas and 'brothel apartments' (*kvartira*), the use of condoms depends on the client. Those who work at train stations or on the street virtually never use them. Little data is available on HIV among prostitutes in the region. However, 10 per cent of female sex workers in Tashkent, Uzbekistan, tested positive in a recent study, and among women who traded drugs for sex, 28 per cent were HIV-infected (Todd *et al.* 2005).

The Soviet system of HIV prevention

Today the HIV epidemic is firmly established in all of the countries of former USSR. Although relatively protected from infection in 1994, the region now has the highest incidence in the world.

HIV went nearly unnoticed in its first years in the USSR, as public authorities and populations faced other, more immediate difficulties. Paradoxically, while most countries in the world were slow in organizing state responses to the coming threat, the Soviet Union quickly implemented a plan of action, despite a then very low infection rate. This system was highly bureaucratic and identical in all parts of the empire, like the rest of the Soviet health system, with uniform training for doctors. As there was no private practice, patients had no options beyond the state health institutions, to which access was tied to their place of residence.

In the mid-1990s this system remained largely in place in the Caucasus and Central Asia. When national governments first requested aid from international agencies, these countries' leaders assumed that the only aid necessary was financial. They did not question the approaches bequeathed by Soviet policy on HIV, including its repressive aspects (Atlani 1998; Atlani *et al.* 2000).

When the first cases of HIV were discovered in the USSR in the mid-1980s, the government and media – in classic Cold War fashion – first blamed the United States. Beginning in October 1985, the Soviet press published numerous articles accusing Washington, the Pentagon and the Centers for Disease Control (CDC) of having created the virus as the first step in a worldwide biological war. To quote *Pravda*: 'The AIDS virus, a terrible disease for which up to now no known cure has been found, was, in the opinion of some Western researchers, created in the laboratories of the Pentagon' (*Pravda*, 31 October 1986, quoted in Williams 1995: 56). 'AIDS was being used as part of Moscow's efforts to discredit the United States by claming the latter was violating the 1935 Geneva Protocol on Chemical Weapons and the 1972 Biological Weapons Convention by engaging in biological warfare activities' (Williams 1995: 56).

Two years later a more pragmatic approach was adopted, though one entirely in line with Soviet ideology. The Supreme Soviet's decree of 25 August 1987 laid out the principal measures to combat the epidemic. First, donors of blood, blood plasma and other biological fluids and tissues were to be tested for HIV; the same also applied to Soviet citizens who had returned from foreign business trips of more than a month's duration. Second, persons in 'high risk groups' (those who had undergone multiple transfusions of blood, drug users, gay men and prostitutes) or Soviet citizens who had had contact with HIV-infected persons were also to be tested. Third, the main means of HIV testing was laboratory blood tests, either voluntarily or during visits to medical institutions. Finally, these new regulations for HIV testing also applied to foreigners on study visits, in employment or to diplomatic and/or consular staff as well as other representatives of international organizations (*Izvestia*, 26 August 1987: 2, quoted in Williams 1995: 58).

In the same year, the Soviet Ministry of Health (*MinZdrav*) created a network of 40 mass testing laboratories for the blood banks and individual testing across the whole of the Soviet territory.

Responsibility for this system was entrusted to the Ministry of Health, which was directly linked to the Communist Party of the Soviet Union. The Ministry's supervision and coordination activities include formulating five-year plans, purchasing medication and equipment, research and development, training of doctors and paramedics, relations with foreign countries, and so on. Operational decisions were assigned to health ministries in the different republics according to the hierarchical structure cascading down through regional health centres, municipalities or districts, and so on.[15] At the top, however, overall policy direction in the fight against the epidemic was provided by the Communist Party of the Soviet Union from 1985 until its formal disappearance in 1991 (see Figure 2.1).

Mass testing[16] and contact tracing[17] were the foundation of the Soviet strategy against HIV. This approach was in force until the fall of the USSR and remained the major point of reference for health personnel in 1995, when the IDO team arrived in the Caucasus and Central Asia (as we shall see).[18] Although Soviet legislation in 1990 guaranteed anonymity in HIV testing, people who were tested often came under strong pressure from governmental organizations still wedded to the practice of contact tracing.

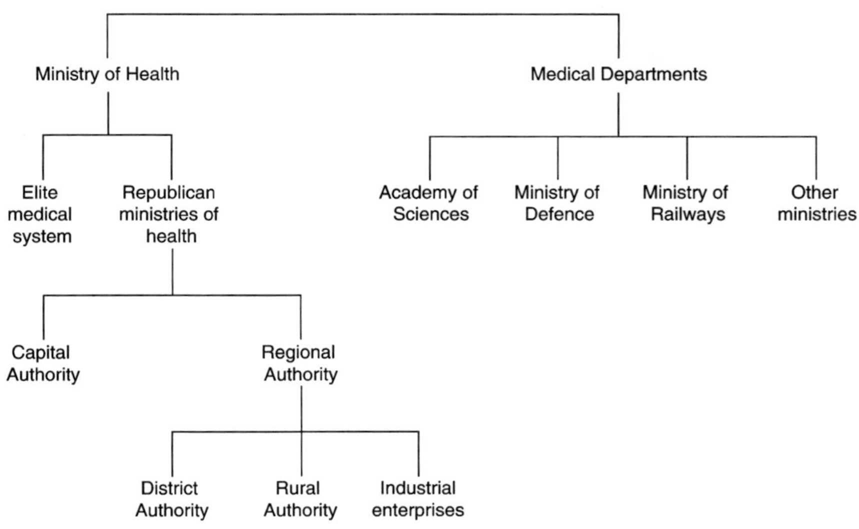

Figure 2.1 The Soviet health system (adapted from Davies 1988: 117).

Unlike in many other parts of the world where non-governmental organizations played major roles in the response to HIV/AIDS, NGOs played no part in the Soviet response. In fact, NGOs in the Western sense of the term were unknown. There were, of course, large numbers of professional, social and cultural organizations, for example labour unions, youth organizations and so on, but they operated under the strict control of the state. In Babajanian's words,

> The existing formal organizations and associations (such as the party, the trade unions, the Young Communist League – *Komsomol*, and others) were controlled by the authoritarian state and were part of the Soviet political structure. Any independent civic associations or activities were seen as a threat to the power of the state.
>
> (Babajanian 2005: 266)

The Soviet constitution had a number of articles concerning voluntary or public associations (*obshestvennie organizatsii*). The 1932 Voluntary Organizations and Associations Act, followed by the 1991 Public Associations Act regulated their creation, activities and conditions of membership. 'Collectivism' was encouraged (Shlapentokh 1989), for example through collective units at work places (Babajanian 2005). But organizations were only authorized if their objectives were in line with those of the state and the Party, and were in effect puppet organizations meant to justify and legitimize official policies. Groups independent of official structures were forbidden (Wedel 1998). As one of my informants put it, 'we risked prison or the *gulag* for any suspicion of illegal association!'

Just before the end of the USSR in 1990 and 1991, some decrees of the Supreme Soviet allowed for the legal creation of independent groups, but their independence was partial and their registration still depended on the state. In Central Asia and the Caucasus, local NGOs developed slowly in the first years following independence, unlike in the other regions of the ex-USSR (notably Russia, Ukraine and the Baltic countries) where local NGOs multiplied, including those working in HIV prevention.

3 Negotiating assistance

As previously noted, by the mid-1990s IDO has decided to provide massive assistance to local NGOs in the region to fight HIV. The decision has two objectives: to prevent the outbreak of an epidemic in the region, and to help improve governance to countries that have just recently received political independence. The IDO actors in this story – unlike those working in the so-called Third World – are new to the region, and have not yet acquired what they consider the necessary know-how to operate there. They are still creating norms and practices for a wide range of aid activities. Although these activities might seem extremely varied, they are rooted in a common approach: the construction of a shared ethos of good governance. Yet this ethos is still theoretical. The actors are being asked to translate it into practice – or more precisely to invent the necessary practices – for a plethora of themes, including HIV prevention in the former Soviet Union.

The actors have arrived at this point convinced that although NGOs may vary in many particulars (for example, in the identities of their members, their activities, hopes, political affiliations, etc.) the form is 'universal'. As the previous chapter showed, however, things are not that simple in the Caucasus and Central Asia. Will the specific conditions and historical context affect the construction of the institutional ideology-in-making? Will they modify it, change its practices? On the contrary: in their search for guidelines permitting them to review or confirm the initial decisions taken in New York, the IDO actors will measure their analyses against the good governance discourse that is increasingly accepted throughout the agency, though the notion is still relatively new and elastic.

Discussion papers from that period reflect this discourse, as well as the actors' awareness that local NGOs in many so-called developing countries are impoverished. 'They lack sufficient capacity in areas such as problem analysis, advocacy and awareness-raising, creation of networks, management, and resource mobilization', says one such paper. 'They need to pay more attention and adapt themselves better to their beneficiaries, and give them more space for involvement in their work. Moreover, some are operating in rigid legal and regulatory environments.' These organizations 'need to build sufficient capacity to reach their full potential' and assume their proper role in good governance. They also need 'an enabling environment within a legal and regulatory framework which guarantees freedom of association, provides the encouragement necessary to facilitate support and administrative processes which permit civil society organizations to take part in the creation and implementation of public policy'.

Within this general framework, according to the official line emanating from headquarters, one of IDO's fundamental tasks in developing countries is to 'bring government and civil society together to talk about policies and programmes, and to create a safe and impartial space which builds confidence and supports the establishment of ongoing relationships'. IDO may also 'support national efforts to review legislative, administrative and fiscal frameworks with a view to reinforcing such organizations, and improving their relationships with state authorities'. Finally, IDO may aim to help these organizations to 'improve their capacity to plan, manage and implement activities in a responsible and effective way'. Where such organizations are almost non-existent, IDO's job is 'to set up the basic institutions of governance'.

Far from letting themselves be daunted by the existing conditions in the post-Soviet Caucasus and Central Asia, and armed with what they consider to be fresh justification for their choices, the IDO actors go in search of anything that might, in one way or another, look like local NGOs with any capacity to fight HIV/AIDS in the region. And if none of them are involved in HIV prevention? 'No problem', say Beth, Anna and their colleagues. 'We'll help them develop the necessary activities.' The IDO actors therefore decide to support a non-existent movement in the fight against the epidemic, despite an existing strategy (i.e., the Soviet approach to HIV control) which is in place but without resources, and which government staff would like to see revived with new funding, including from international sources.

Supporting local NGOs doing HIV prevention is only one aspect of IDO's multi-faceted approach to the epidemic in the region. IDO is also working on reform and improvement of HIV testing procedures, respect for anonymity and confidentiality, provision of psycho-social support, and HIV-awareness campaigns appropriate for vulnerable groups, as well as better treatment of sexually transmitted diseases and access to care for people living with HIV/AIDS. The support provided to local HIV-prevention NGOs in the name of promoting good governance is only part of IDO's wider work.

This phase in the construction of an institutional ideology advances in three stages. First, the IDO actors undertake strong advocacy in favour of action through local NGOs, aimed at the only actors currently responding to HIV/AIDS in the region: government officials. Second, they attempt to make contact with all forms of organizations, identified as NGOs or not, which might one day develop non-governmental activities for HIV prevention. These organizations fall into three types: rebaptized institutions of the former Soviet Union, recently created NGOs and what the IDO actors call 'nascent NGOs'. Third, and last, IDO deploys a concrete strategy of support for the local NGOs that have been identified. As the years pass, this international support will be elaborated around two key approaches: material and technical assistance to local NGOs, and promotion of the legislative and social framework necessary for their development. The goal is to permit the flowering of civil society – a civil society composed of the local NGOs which are supposed to be the guarantors of good governance.

Advocacy

To begin with, the IDO staff set themselves the task of convincing government actors that a new approach is the correct one. Beyond the rhetoric of official documents that uniformly tout 'the need for civil society' in these countries, this advocacy is carried out in conversations and small group discussions which are later taken up in villages, *rayon* (district) headquarters and capital cities. With it, the IDO actors arrive at a new stage of dialogue (which includes confrontations, occasionally stressful ones) with government officials who still cleave to the established political 'line'. Apart from mass testing and contact tracing, there have been a few additional prevention activities, such as HIV/AIDS education and information. Some products were designed and produced between 1987 and 1991, including posters, badges, stickers and brochures following the STI prevention model. But these were never a priority in Soviet times, when the focus was on mass testing and surveillance of individuals suspected of 'bad lifestyles'.

This one-track approach to the epidemic, a legacy of both the recent past and the longer social history of the Soviet Union, is the response that Beth, Anna, Lena, Igor and their IDO colleagues frequently receive from their interlocutors when they describe the type of assistance they hope to provide to requesting countries. In fact, their advocacy for 'mobilization' of local NGOs provokes unease among the health administrators and professionals, most of whom are still state officials.

It is winter in one of the small towns of a former Soviet republic in Central Asia. The meeting is underway in the offices of the Ministry of Health. The huge room is unheated, with a bone-chilling dampness in the air. Thick orange and maroon curtains, faded green and yellow paint on the walls, plywood tables and chairs, three light fixtures hanging from the ceiling: everything is redolent of the 1950s, a mixture of austerity and administrative rigidity that simultaneously evokes the classroom, the hospital and the barracks. Added to this is the indefinable but unmistakable atmosphere – slightly suffocating – so characteristic of the bureaucratic world spawned by Soviet society during its time as a world power.

Beth, Anna, Lena and Igor represent IDO at this meeting. As we have seen, Beth and Anna are expatriates new to the region, while Lena and Igor are local IDO employees, nationals of the country like the other participants. The latter, judged by their clothes, appear to be a homogeneous group.

All are bundled up in heavy coats and fur hats. In fact, they are highly diverse. The majority are doctors, nurses and paramedics from the Ministry of Health, but there are also veterans of organizations resuscitated from Soviet times, representatives of the prison service and the teams responsible for surveillance of 'drug addicts' and 'prostitutes', doctors from family planning centres, and the director of a public clinic for sexually transmitted infections.

While Beth and her colleagues once again describe the urgent issues that need to be addressed, a couple of men chat aside from the others (like the other dialogues and debates in this book, the following is reconstructed from notes I made at the time).

SERGEI: 'Tell me, Oleg, have you any idea why we're here?'

OLEG (*pulling out the letter of invitation and summarizing it ironically*): 'To learn how we and our institutions can adapt ourselves to the guidelines promised by the international agencies that have come to help us.'

SERGEI (*none the wiser*): 'I see . . .'

BETH (*speaking to the group*): 'As you all know, syphilis and prostitution are spreading in your region, and there is little use of condoms. Drug trafficking is rising steadily and an increasing number of young people are becoming addicted. The HIV virus is knocking at the region's gate! If you are going to prevent an epidemic, both the state and local NGOs will need to get involved.'

A PARTICIPANT (*astonished, as is the rest of the group*): 'Tell me, what is a local NGO?'

IGOR: 'NGOs are people like you, who got organized in order to tackle problems that the government can't deal with alone.'

A PARTICIPANT: 'The government has no money. Our salaries haven't been paid for two years!'

ANOTHER PARTICIPANT: 'Back in Soviet times, we had lots of organizations. Women's organizations, youth organizations, factory workers unions, sport associations, chess players, *oblast* committees, ethnic minorities and cultural groups. . . . They're all gone now.'

BETH: 'Those were all extensions of the Communist Party, and they did what they were told. That's not what we mean by civil society. I'm talking about non-governmental organizations, meaning *in-de-pen-dent* ones.' (*Heavy silence ensues.*) 'Civil society is one of the central pillars of good governance, and local NGOs are one of the main ingredients.'

IGOR (*breaking a silence as long and heavy as the previous one*): 'It is absolutely vital that NGOs be part of the fight against HIV/AIDS. I can see that most of you are doctors and that you work for the state. Well, preventing this epidemic will need a more nuanced approach than purely state or medical interventions, which is all we have in this region at the moment.'

A THIRD PARTICIPANT (*both plaintive and a little hostile*): 'Before, all medical problems were looked after by state health centres. But they don't have any resources these days. It has been months since the doctors have been paid. So now, if I understand correctly, the epidemic is supposed to be dealt with by others?[1] By non-doctors – and therefore non-professionals – and by marginal groups?'

A FOURTH: 'If they only had adequate funding, the health centres could continue to do mass testing and surveillance of deviant individuals. Then the infected people could easily be identified and controlled, just like in the USSR.'

Beth reiterates the necessity of breaking with the practices of Soviet times, and emphasizes that it is no longer a question of identifying and controlling individuals but of preventing an epidemic – a task that local NGOs are better placed to carry out than the state health services.

BETH: 'International experience is conclusive about this. Civil society groups understand the population and its needs. They can talk about delicate issues, about sexuality and other behaviours that government services can't deal with. You need individuals talking to individuals, women talking to women, HIV-positive people talking with other HIV-positive people, drug users talking to other drug users . . .'

A television journalist is present in the room, since this is the first time that a non-medical international development agency has undertaken a major HIV/AIDS initiative in the region. He is amazed by what he is hearing.

THE JOURNALIST: 'Is this really so urgent? Remember, HIV is hardly present in our country, and there are no local NGOs working in this field.'

LENA: 'That's why we're here. You need to listen to what we're saying!'

ANNA: 'This is the ideal time to act. There are very few cases of HIV so far. But there are some worrying signs like the rise of STIs. We know from experience that an HIV epidemic can explode very quickly. So it's very important that different actors, including local NGOs, are aware of the problem and participate in the prevention work.'

BETH (*trying to explain IDO's intentions*): 'We're not here to dictate what people have to do. For the moment all we are here to do is spend some time with representatives of government and civil society, learn about the situation, and put our heads together about how IDO can help. After that, we plan to provide assistance for a limited period of time, putting funding and technical resources at the disposal of governments and local NGOs in the region, if the latter are created and decide to get involved in the fight against the epidemic.'

IGOR: 'First and foremost, we'll assist emerging civil society organizations to develop activities and get in contact with American or European counterparts who've already been working against the epidemic for a number of years.'

When the long meeting ends, it is almost night. Sergei and his colleagues, whom the people from the agency doubt they have convinced, break open some Soviet champagne before moving on to cognac, and then to vodka.

There are two reasons for this group's unease. The first is the governmental context inherited from the Soviet Union, which explains the quasi-absence of local NGOs and the rigidly structured government strategies for fighting HIV/AIDS, all of them based on a single model. The second stems from the conditions in which administrative authority in the newly independent republics has found itself since the fall of the USSR: 'abandoned' – at least that is the perception of the majority of government actors – and cut off from the orders, guidelines, information, funding and technical assistance of the old days.

The following extract from a discussion illustrates this mixture of incomprehension and suspicion. It occurs in Vladimir's office between Anna, Beth, Igor, Lena and Vladimir, who is the state secretary for AIDS in the region (he has the same position as Eldar in a neighbouring country). Vladimir is surrounded by his main colleagues, all of them civil servants. The office is a modest one in a building belonging to the Ministry of Health. The walls are covered in books and annotated documents, with HIV prevention posters tacked up here and there. People come and go ceaselessly, bundled up against the cold, bringing papers for signature.

ANNA: 'Our project focuses on support for good governance, specifically among local NGOs. We want to show you some models from successful HIV/AIDS initiatives in other countries.'

VLADIMIR: 'The Western countries offer us assistance. Yet they themselves have very high levels of HIV infection . . . So their approaches don't seem so effective to me! Forgive me, maybe I'm just an ignorant doctor stuck in a corner of an empire that no longer exists, but what are these new prevention experiences that are supposed to inspire us?'

BETH: 'In some countries, people organized groups to work within their communities doing HIV prevention and caring for people living with the disease.'

VLADIMIR: 'Maybe the epidemic has been sent to put fear into people and force them to act more responsibly. If God didn't exist, we'd have to invent Him!'

BETH: 'What can you tell me about local NGOs doing HIV prevention?'

VLADIMIR: 'There aren't any NGOs doing prevention here, so obviously we haven't been working with them. But we do have numerous social institutions that are involved.'

IGOR: 'Might they be interested in technical assistance and training in methods being used elsewhere?'

VLADIMIR: 'Sure, why not?'

AN ASSISTANT: 'NGOs are a new idea for us. Their work is also new . . .'

ANNA: 'Yes, that's understood. After a half century of Soviet power in which government was the only provider of services, there isn't a favourable context for non-governmental activities. Establishing local NGOs won't be easy.'

BETH: 'And of course, the epidemic is still considered a medical problem to be managed by state institutions . . . That doesn't help either, does it?'

A COLLEAGUE: 'Er, well . . . So, what are local NGOs like, in the rest of the world?'

LENA: 'Let the experts speak!'

ANNA (*gently defusing the tension*): 'They are groups of people who get together with the goal of dealing collectively with their own problems and aspirations. They don't expect the government to do it for them or to tell them what to do. Local NGOs have been very useful in the fight against HIV in many countries. For example, some parts of the population are beginning to protect themselves, even though they didn't feel that official prevention campaigns had anything to do with them.'

IGOR: 'The responses developed around the world during the past ten years have produced some successful models and guidelines. Experience suggests that without the strong presence of local NGOs and involved communities, it is very difficult to halt the epidemic's advance. In both developed and developing countries, local NGOs are actually the principal actors in the fight against HIV/AIDS.'

A COLLEAGUE: 'In concrete terms, what do they actually do?'

BETH: 'Some do awareness-building among their own communities about the dangers of infection and strategies for avoiding it. Others work to reduce the suspicion that surrounds the disease, and the fear it sometimes provokes. They may help find places for HIV-positive people to live if they've been rejected by their family and friends. Or make sure that these people have access to certain types of treatment, and that it is delivered in good conditions . . . Those are just a few examples.'

VLADIMIR: 'And in concrete terms, what is the goal of your project?'

ANNA: 'We're here to help local NGOs develop programmes for prevention of HIV. That will be done through technical and financial assistance to existing local NGOs that want to create their own prevention activities, and to individuals who want to create local NGOs with HIV prevention as their primary goal.'

A COLLEAGUE: 'What you ought to be doing is helping us revive our own system instead of helping marginal groups who aren't even professionals. *We* are professionals; our health system used to be excellent. But we don't even get our salaries any more. And everything has to be paid for . . . So here you are, come to help drug addicts and homosexuals! Which don't even exist here! And they're illegal. We send people like that to prison! How are they supposed to help protect the population against AIDS? This isn't Africa, you know!'

A COLLEAGUE: 'Look, we haven't been paid in months. Our testing equipment is old, from Soviet times, and we don't have the money to replace parts that wear out . . . Maybe local NGOs would be better than what we have now.'

A COLLEAGUE: 'Why don't we just create an NGO within our ministry!'

LENA (*seriously*): 'That's right, you have to listen to us if you want a future.'

IGOR (*uncomfortably*): 'Fine, but . . . well . . . It's just that we're supposed to be helping NGOs, meaning *non*-governmental organizations.'

ANNA: 'Also, we'll help those who have a clear idea of their objectives and target populations, so long as they've developed a proper detailed work plan. They need to be fully committed to respect for human rights. As the government's Centre for AIDS, you are in a good position to collaborate with local NGOs . . .'

BETH: 'But it is really important that the members of local NGOs aren't simultaneously representatives of the state. That would be contrary to the desired objective.'

VLADIMIR: 'But what is that objective?'

IGOR: 'Why, to create an active civil society that cooperates with representatives of the state like you but isn't under your control.'

It is important to note that this initial incomprehension (sometimes mixed with hostility), when public health officials first encounter IDO and its projects, is not an isolated event that is only seen in the corridors of power, but is shared by the majority of professionals. Later on, as we will see, some will adopt the development agency's vision. For the moment, however, in the mid-1990s, they make no effort to hide their scepticism about the proposals made to them, while at the same time confessing how lost they feel in this still astonishing post-Soviet world. In fact, the IDO actors are rapidly confronted with the fact that the fall of the Soviet system has left a large majority of health professionals in real confusion about the HIV epidemic. The government departments in each newly independent country have been cut off from the supervision and planning of the Ministry of Health (*MinZdrav*) in Moscow; suddenly, they have to decide on their own policies and practices to face the epidemic, at a time when the dismantling of the health system has interrupted their access to information. As the IDO representatives noticed when they arrived, the majority of the region's health professionals are now out of touch what is happening outside their country.

Beginning in 1995, this advocacy in favour of local NGOs and their role in fighting HIV/AIDS takes the form – especially in the early days – of information, much of it almost polemical, as we have seen in the previous chapter. From 1997, it accelerates and reaches the most isolated provinces as the years pass. The discourse and practices of the IDO actors take on a stability and coherence, informed both by documented experiences of HIV/AIDS-oriented NGOs in the West and by increasing knowledge of post-Soviet conditions and actors, and of their logic and practices. The following extracts illustrate this evolution and the patient work of explication it involved. What stands out is that this advocacy is presented as 'technical', implying that it is scientific and politically neutral, even though in fact it is a mix of different levels of discourse.

A winter's evening in 1998, in a small city which is the administrative centre of an isolated mountain province. Beth, Anna and Olozbiek are having a meeting. Olozbiek works in a state clinic and is in charge of STI and HIV prevention in the province. The night is black because the street-lights have not been working for two years, due to a lack of funding. The facades of the Soviet-style apartment blocks are dilapidated. Only the young and the *babushkas* go outdoors, where it is six below zero. We are spending the evening in one of the city's few restaurants, with its disco-style decor so characteristic of the post-Soviet republics. The room is dark and almost empty, with mirrored balls hanging from the ceiling. A musical ensemble plays on a podium – a synthesizer player and a guitarist in suits from the 1970s, and a young woman singer. They play the latest Russian and Turkish hits. Groups of bored girls and women sit at tables around the edges of the dance floor. As for us, we sit in a small, windowless side-room with sliding doors, off the main room of the disco/restaurant.

Today, as on so many other occasions since the programme began (though with different interlocutors), Beth is lambasting the punitive measures implemented by post-Soviet governments to hold back the epidemic, while Olozbiek defends them. Beth cannot understand what such measures are supposed to accomplish, and invokes the right to anonymity and respect for people living with HIV/AIDS, their families and the other people in their lives. This is not the first time we have heard this debate on discrimination against people affected by the epidemic, a debate played out in other parts of the former Soviet Union. The pattern has been seen before in many countries where HIV has revealed itself. It has been characterized as attempts by governments, in the name of health considerations, to reassert control over 'marginal' groups and 'at-risk' individuals, as if they can be separated from the general population and the world of politics.[2] As we have seen in previous chapters, the legacy of Soviet public health policies against HIV/AIDS is still heavily in evidence.

OLOZBIEK: 'You say that vulnerable groups need to be able to organize themselves against the epidemic. But what about the rights of society in general?'

ANNA: 'What you're suggesting is that there are two competing interests: the interests of HIV-positive people and those of everyone else. . . . They had this same debate in other countries back at the beginning of the epidemic.'

OLOZBIEK: 'Our Soviet system was based on this idea of competing interests and the necessity of choosing between them. We happen to think that the primary interest should be the health of society in general . . .'

BETH: '... which under the Soviet regime justified all sorts of discriminatory measures that ignored the rights of people with sexually transmitted diseases or HIV ...'

OLOZBIEK: 'You can't deny that there are conflicting interests! We don't understand why, in the West, you don't isolate infected people from everyone else. People who endanger society should be removed from the rest of the population. That's how we used to do it in the USSR. The state was responsible for individuals, not the other way round.' (*He continues his train of thought.*) 'Western logic can be difficult to conceptualize in the Soviet context. Our idea of responsibility was different. The only responsibility was that of the state for the good of the collective.'

ANNA: 'It doesn't have to be seen as a conflict. The moment one sees a conflict between the health of society on one side and the rights of HIV-positive people on the other, there is a subtext of "them" and "us". As if "we" will never be at risk of infection or be close to someone affected by the epidemic ... It just isn't true.'

OLOZBIEK: 'But "we" need to protect ourselves. And that means staying in the "we" zone ...'

BETH: 'Yes, "we" can choose to protect ourselves, but sometimes we're vulnerable, some of us more than others. Which means our choices regarding HIV can be either helped or hindered by certain factors in our environment.'[3]

OLOZBIEK: 'Can you give me an example of these "factors"?'

BETH: 'In some groups, for example, using a condom is easy to do because safe sex is part of that group's mores. In others, it is much harder to insist that a partner use one. So the latter are more vulnerable than the former ...'

ANNA: 'The economic situation can also be a factor of vulnerability. In general, and in the way most of us live our daily lives, it can limit our capacity to choose ...'[4] (*with a look towards the main room where young girls in heavy makeup are dancing – the proprietor offered us their company when we arrived*) 'There are also people who are forced to do certain types of work, by economic circumstances for example, that make them vulnerable to HIV. The most obvious one is prostitution. Prostitutes are not always able to insist that their clients use condoms.'

BETH: 'Another example that you often find in this region relates to the link between STIs and HIV. You know better than I how difficult it has become to treat STIs since the fall of the Soviet Union. True, if one wants to get treatment, there is a lot more choice than before. But the economic situation and the general disorganization of the system put the whole population in a situation of vulnerability!' (*Here Beth stops herself and returns to Olozbiek's question*): 'All of which means that this period of political and economic transition here in the former USSR has multiplied the factors of vulnerability to HIV/AIDS ... and one of the responses to that vulnerability is a civil society that is strong in relation to the government.'

The evening ends hours later, after numerous toasts with vodka. The following are extracts from a number of different conversations. Again, the discussions are familiar to IDO staff members, who have had time to refine their arguments since 1995.

OLOZBIEK: 'Last night at the restaurant you talked about factors of vulnerability to HIV in this country. But how are we to modify these factors?'

BETH: 'Individuals acting on their own can't bring all the changes necessary to reduce those factors. Certainly, they have to take responsibility and try to protect themselves from HIV, but they need help from their surrounding environment in order to have the capacity to exercise that responsibility. That's where civil society organizations have a role. They are essential to creating an environment that is open, tolerant and non-discriminatory, and to supporting the most vulnerable and helping them access HIV prevention programmes.'

A PARTICIPANT FROM A LOCAL WOMEN'S NGO: 'You mean like support for people who are infected.'

ANNA: 'Right, that's an example. A lot of HIV-positive people may not be able to reveal their sero-status, or are afraid to find out, because of the environment they live in.'

OLOZBIEK: 'Are you suggesting we discriminate in favour of NGOs for infected people? On the contrary, the state should be taking measures to ensure that those people aren't infecting other people on purpose! Like during Soviet times!'

ANNA (*heatedly*): 'And if that happened, what makes you think that the victims of such measures would care about protecting themselves or protecting others? What means would they have to do so? They'd be on their own, with no emotional or material support that might help them act as responsible participants in the fight against HIV.'

BETH: 'HIV-prevention activities can be stymied by a hostile governmental environment, where people can't talk openly about their behaviour or discuss the risks they face. By that I mean the environment left over from the Soviet Union.'

ANNA: 'If we're going to prevent the epidemic here, certain factors of vulnerability will have to be addressed. And that can't be done by government services alone; they aren't representative of civil society. That's why local NGOs are essential.'

A GOVERNMENT REPRESENTATIVE: 'You say that our governments don't represent the people. But they are elected!'

BETH: 'That's right, they are elected. But you need an ongoing countervailing power to the state. Just because a government is elected doesn't ensure it will respect its commitments, its laws, or the rights of citizens ... [5] A strong civil society is a counter-power which allows non-democratic excesses to be avoided.'

A MEMBER OF A LOCAL STUDENTS' ASSOCIATION: 'Do you think NGOs are strong enough to do all that?'

BETH: 'Maybe not yet. Maybe it's still a bit early, given the Soviet history you've inherited. It's true that NGOs here aren't very strong yet. But it will come. You'll need to create that relationship between isolated individuals and the state if you want to avoid the return of a totalitarian regime . . . If civil society becomes strong enough to influence the state, it will help to move forward the political and economic reforms your countries have been attempting to carry out since the fall of the USSR.'

A PARTICIPANT: 'Are those reforms really worth defending?'

BETH: 'You are in a period of transition. Things are tough, and that's why you aren't sure it's worth it. But do you want to go back to a totalitarian regime?'

A PARTICIPANT (*laughing*): 'We've strayed a long way from AIDS, haven't we?'

BETH: 'Actually, not that far! That's exactly why our project promotes the role of NGOs here – to fight the epidemic, and by doing so build the institutions needed for good governance.'

In search of partners

Along with their advocacy with the government professionals in favour of a role for local NGOs in fighting the epidemic, the IDO staff members are looking out for any local organizations that might eventually develop non-state HIV prevention activities, even if they are not (for the moment) involved in such work or even calling themselves 'local NGOs'.

The first ones are former Soviet associations that have been rebaptized as NGOs. While many associations and mass organizations disappeared after the fall of the USSR, others survived in new forms, often taken in hand by young professionals and white-collar workers (Wedel 1998). Large entities with considerable experience and many contacts, they are more attuned to responding to the expectations of higher authorities than the needs of the 'base'. Impelled by some of their members, some have turned themselves into true private enterprises that are perfectly comfortable with financial negotiations. The NGO Dynamic Youth is a good example. During Soviet times it was the national branch of the Communist Union of Youth (*Komsomol*), to which a large number of adolescents and young adults belonged – mostly due to social and ideological pressure rather than conviction. It still shows signs of life in the aftermath of independence, which is visible in its headquarters. The 400,000 members of the old association are still on its books, though it recognizes that only two thousand of them are really 'activists'. The building is well appointed. Above the portico at the entrance to the building hangs – as in Soviet times but with new colours – a flag bearing the emblem of the newly independent country. On the desks are baskets of metallic pins bearing the same emblem and the logo of the 'new' association. One of the current directors was on the governing board of the *Komsomol* during its transformation into an NGO. This allowed him to travel to many international youth conferences and gain familiarity with the international development agencies now arriving in the country. His clothes are well cut, and he is a director of many private companies.

One senses that his attitude to the fight against HIV/AIDS is divided between the old procedures, which he considers just and effective, and the need to take heed of the proposals of the IDO actors, whose financial resources are of no small interest to his organization. His assistant prompts him with a whispered list of prevention activities that are (supposedly) being done by his NGO.

THE DIRECTOR (*enumerating them*): 'Propaganda, information posters for schools, organizing a sports marathon . . .'

IGOR (*recognizing the list as directly lifted from Soviet HIV/AIDS programming*): 'Have these actually been implemented by your organization?'

THE DIRECTOR (*evasive*): 'Well, you might say some are in various stages of planning, or in preparation for the implementation stages.'

BETH: 'Do your activities deal directly with drug use? With addiction? With HIV prevention among injecting drug users?'

THE DIRECTOR (*indignant*): 'We're not the mafia! We don't work with marginal groups! Our HIV prevention activities are very professional!'

IGOR: 'What HIV prevention activities would your NGO like to implement?'

THE ASSISTANT: 'Er, well, we've come up with some ideas and we plan to . . .'

THE DIRECTOR (*smoothly*): 'We're going to create an anti-AIDS committee and come up with an action plan! But, in the words of Napoleon, "it takes money to make war". So, what are you proposing to fund us to do? What type of programme do you want us to set up?'

BETH: 'In order to create prevention activities that are adapted to existing conditions, one needs to analyse the hopes and expectations of the people involved, the beneficiaries of the support. We don't have any predetermined plans. It's up to you to create the activities of your choice. As representatives of civil society, you are closer to the population than we are. That's why the participation of NGOs like yours is so essential. You know what will make young people respond, what they'll think and what they'll do. We don't have any intention of dictating what you ought to be doing – quite the contrary.'

THE DIRECTOR (*suddenly looking at Beth and Igor with suspicion*): 'Are there any programmes that IDO has funded elsewhere in the world that have worked well?'

BETH: 'Certainly. This approach to NGOs has been tried successfully in a number of countries in Latin America, Asia and Africa.'

THE DIRECTOR: 'But those are under-developed countries! We're the ones who educated their professionals! They used to come to study here in our Soviet universities.'

BETH: 'Obviously, there are enormous cultural, social, political and economic differences between one country and another. That's precisely why we are asking you to describe what you intend to do, and how you intend to do it.'

THE DIRECTOR: 'The members of our association are highly qualified people. Tell us what you want us to do, and it will be done with total professionalism! If you can clearly state what you want, we can deliver. Just give us your plan!'

The responses from other members of Dynamic Youth are more moderate. They say they are ready to try new approaches to prevention. But they still ask for a plan. 'We're totally open to other ways of doing things', they say. 'If you could just tell us how Western NGOs usually proceed, we'll change our methods. But we need information and new ideas . . . We are just so used to having others tell us what to do.'

It would be incorrect to interpret the different behaviours of the director and these colleagues as a confrontation of 'old guard' and 'new guard'. Even those who say they are ready to build new prevention services do not hide their discomfort at having to work alongside groups of addicts or homosexuals. And in both cases – old guard and those who have put on new clothes – one observes the same incomprehension when faced with the IDO staff, these apparent 'experts' who nonetheless offer no ready-made plans for the NGO to implement. The fact that the funder has no plan to impose is difficult for these Soviet-trained 'community' actors to understand, and seems to them lacking in the professionalism to which they are so attached.

As they systematically search for actors capable of carrying out effective prevention activities, Beth, Igor, Anna and their colleagues discover other members of the new generation – this time, people who have created NGOs that are the offspring of government structures. Their members do not come from defunct Soviet associations, as is the case with Dynamic Youth, but from governmental institutions such as medical institutes, family planning units and the medico-legal departments that dealt with drug addiction. Their creation reflects international conditions, with some having decided to transform themselves into NGOs expressly in order to attract external finance.

As we have seen, independence was accompanied by a drastic cutback in health budgets. In the early years, salaries were no longer paid, medicines were lacking and the staff were demoralized. Some institutions officially became NGOs, often retaining their state identity while receiving significant international funding. Their members, if specialized in a field such as family planning, are regularly invited to international conferences or training on contraception or psychological support for patients. Nonetheless, their practices and their visions of prevention and care reveal to the IDO members that here too, in the mid-1990s, the NGO dimension is still no more than a change of costume.[6]

The NGO Women Together came out of the Institute of Gynaecology and Obstetrics, another legacy of the Soviet family planning system. The members of the NGO are all doctors or paramedics on the staff of the Institute – in other words, civil servants hired during the Soviet era. For two years they have received financial support from a number of international development agencies in the field of family planning. The walls of their meeting room bear proof of this: they are festooned with documents and posters in English, singing the praises of the pill.

THE NGO DIRECTOR: 'What we do is family planning. We receive five thousand women per year, of whom a large number (40 per cent of patients who come for a check-up) have a sexually transmitted infection, particularly syphilis. Examinations and care are delivered within an overall framework of general gynaecology, pregnancy, infertility and abortion. The team has recently started prescribing the pill and IUDs. We'd be delighted to receive your funding!'

MIKE (*letting the last remark pass*): 'What about condoms?'

A DOCTOR: 'We don't advise people to use condoms. We talk about them if people ask, that's all. You see, our mandate here is contraception.'

BETH (*astonished*): 'I'm not sure I understand your reasoning. STIs are on the rise – why do you think that is?'

ANOTHER STAFF MEMBER: 'Because of the decline in morality!'

A DOCTOR: 'Luckily, certain prostitutes come to see us once a month. They are sent by their pimp, who pays for treatment if they have an STI.'

ANNA: 'But there is no treatment for HIV!'

THE DIRECTOR (*categorically*): 'We haven't had any cases of HIV so far, so there is no problem!'

In the face of this straightforward denial of the existence of HIV in the region, Mike gives a long description of the Latin American experience, where groups of women have formed NGOs to raise awareness among other women about HIV's existence and how to prevent it. They carry out information activities in the street, in hospital waiting rooms and so on. These NGOs also provide a space for women to talk freely about subjects such as STIs, HIV and sexual relations with their partners. These activities have seen significant results in prevention, says Mike.

THE DIRECTOR (*interrupting Mike, condescendingly*): 'Obviously they are doing some interesting things down there ... But here, 100 per cent of women have finished school. Unlike in South America, they aren't dependent on their husbands. Almost all are working. And believe me, the Soviet system taught them to take responsibility for themselves!'

Although expressed differently, the reaction of the director of this NGO and many of her colleagues is analogous to that of the director of Dynamic

Youth. Both consist of a vehement protest and a refusal that this place, its personnel and the majority of women attended here should be confused in any way with some exotic 'under-developed country'. They proudly describe the quality of information given in the 'counselling centres' created since the Soviet period in the country's public health clinics, and the value of the information meetings run by health professionals.

A NURSE: 'This high level of professionalism is widely recognized. For instance, the police give us their list of women at risk, particularly prostitutes. We make sure they all come to see us, even if forcing them to do so can be difficult.'

MIKE: 'You think using police methods to control populations for reasons of public health is professional? No, what you need is a non-governmental approach, based on the free choice of individuals and guaranteed anonymity.'

THE NURSE: 'Well, we've tried to organize public information meetings, but no one comes.'

MIKE: 'That's quite possibly *because* you are an official medical institution. I was talking about the work of NGOs.'

The dialogue is going nowhere, and the director wraps up, her studied smile totally gone: 'Women don't have time for this type of discussion. Time is money!' Anna, Beth and Mike are just as ready to leave. Their hopes of finding partners with a spirit of public service or empathy with the people who eventually will turn up HIV-positive, rather than the obvious distaste shown so far, are being slowly ground into dust.

Clearly, for a large number of Government Organized NGOs (or GONGOs) that have come out of institutions inherited from the Soviet period, the new label has not changed much in their management practices or the way they care for their 'beneficiaries'. Although extreme, this example permits some appreciation of the difficulties in communication between IDO staff and the members of this type of NGO. With a style of management and an approach to HIV prevention copied directly from the Soviet model, on the one hand, and an influx of funds from the international development agencies (in this case from their family planning programmes) on the other, in the mid-1990s these NGOs still have not fundamentally questioned what they do and how they do it.

Unlike the old Soviet institutions and associations that have been rebaptized as NGOs, the second type of collective group that Igor, Beth and their IDO colleagues are contacting include newly created local NGOs that have no relation to any official structures. They include small organizations that have been created recently in the mid-1990s, and whose founders are attempting to use the post-Soviet freedoms to turn their dreams into action. They are of modest size, and so far somewhat ill defined, due to their being 'works in progress'. One NGO can be used to illustrate the type.

Somewhat extreme in their idealism, the members of the NGO Sexuality and Pleasure are not active in HIV/AIDS when Beth, Igor and Anna come to visit, but are starting to work in the related field of sexuality. Beth, Igor and Anna have contacted them in hopes that they might be able to extend their activities to include HIV prevention. They have their first meeting in the basement of a school. The organization is composed of three individuals in their 40s: Atkan, a male high school teacher who is the NGO's director, and two women, a social worker named Vera and a journalist named Ludmilla. The three got together barely a year ago with the objectives of publishing a magazine and providing public forums on sexuality. Sitting in the classroom, the three friends – wearing thick glasses and turtle-neck sweaters, cigarettes in hand – diffidently take turns explaining their project.

ATKAN: 'We aren't used to talking about our activities, or rather, our projects. We haven't met with any foreigners yet, and we haven't really looked for funding. But we've heard you might be able to help us.'

VERA: 'For the moment, we've spent most of our time sorting out the paperwork needed to become a legal NGO. Some friends have donated the money to rent this room once a week and prepare to publish our magazine.'

LUDMILLA: 'We want to talk about sexuality and pleasure, relations with couples, homosexuality, bisexuality . . .'

ATKAN (*with an embarrassed smile*): 'You know, these are subjects you couldn't bring up publicly in the past, at least officially . . . And that hasn't really changed.'

Beth and Anna are taken with these newcomers with their genuine interest in exploring issues of human sexuality. Beth doubts that they will survive, given their obvious inexperience at marketing themselves and their lack of understanding both of international donor logic and the Byzantine intrigues of the ministries. Anna agrees for the most part, but insists that they be included in planned training exercises to give them a fighting chance.

This NGO is typical of a certain number of non-state associations born in the first years of independence: modest, inexperienced in managing collective efforts and composed of members who are driven by ideas that they are trying to turn into reality, so far without much success. Lost in the new, post-Soviet world, they are trying to make use of the relative liberty of association that has opened up, but are not sure how to do so. They have not learned even the basics of managing an organization – public or private, governmental or associative – or the new 'rules of the game' that NGOs such as Dynamic Youth have mastered perfectly.

The other extreme among the recently formed NGOs encountered by the IDO team is visible in an organization called Active Women, whose activities are guided primarily by the profit motive. This NGO was created by women, mostly from the wealthier class, who have put together a project similar to Françoise Dolto's *Maison Verte* nurturing centres. The idea is to offer women a welcoming space where they will be listened to and can receive all kinds of information about sexuality, couple relations and child education. But although the clients can receive information and counselling for free, they will also be able to buy the pill – in a country where, it should be remembered, abortion is still widely used as contraception.

Though initially impressed by their dynamism, the IDO team rapidly realize that this organization's ethical framework regarding HIV prevention is still that of the Soviet era, rooted in the practices of identifying and condemning people deemed to be 'a danger to society as a whole'. Another characteristic of this NGO – like many others of its type – is that it receives funding from large foreign companies operating in the country (particularly those interested in its oil and gas resources) and is close to international pharmaceutical companies producing oral contraceptives. Such companies have been exploring opportunities in the region, which they consider an 'emerging market' for the historical reasons discussed in the previous chapter. Since they are in the business of selling the pill (as well as providing free advice), the members of this NGO consider condoms – despite the protection they provide against HIV – to be in competition with oral contraceptives. As a result, they are more interested in revenue from selling the pill than in distributing condoms, in line with their international pharmaceutical partners. There are many such groups which are attempting to surf the wave of post-Soviet transition and which, despite calling themselves NGOs and being legally registered as such, are in reality private businesses (Berg 2003). With the number of associations independent of the state emerging, and certain gaps in the relevant legislation, it is easy for a profit-based entity to call itself an NGO.

Somewhere between these two extremes – modest, idealistic groups such as Sexuality and Pleasure, and extensions of commercial enterprise such as Active Women – can be found an NGO called Boda, which though recently created and small in size, is confident of future success and funding. Boda has two important characteristics: its goal is HIV prevention (even if it has not implemented any activities so far) and its director is an *apparatchik* who was a specialist in HIV control during the Soviet era.

Tatiana is a doctor. She was originally a high official in the Ministry of Health and became state secretary for AIDS, but had to leave her post at the beginning of the 1990s – 'for corruption' say her detractors, particularly Eldar, who replaced her. It is impossible to know whether the charge is well founded or the result of personal animosity, a struggle for influence between two formerly eminent actors in the Soviet-era health system who were trained in the same methods. During a working meeting at the state secretariat, one of the IDO members mentions Boda as evidence that 'things are going in the right direction', and that 'initiatives are beginning to emerge from civil society'. Eldar violently denigrates Boda (and particularly its director), charging that the NGO has no real contacts among HIV-positive people – a monopoly he claims for himself. His words are blunt: 'That organization doesn't know a single infected person! Its members have no idea who is infected. I'm the only one who knows! I'm in charge of AIDS in this country. No one else knows the names of the infected people, because we respect anonymity!'

Clearly, he cannot stand the idea that Tatiana considers herself still active in the response to HIV/AIDS. He declares without embarrassment that he wants to be the 'only boss of the epidemic'.

Nonetheless, Tatiana has indeed created her little NGO, and she is at once Boda's president and only truly active member. Later on, she is joined by her son and some of his student friends. Beth, Mike, Anna and their colleagues meet her during their ongoing search for potential civil society partners, and are surprised to find that even before IDO has begun any activities in the country, Tatiana is well aware of international experience in the fight against HIV/AIDS, including the importance of NGOs in the response. During her time as state secretary, she was regularly invited to international HIV/AIDS conferences, and understands the West's approach. In practice, however, the IDO team becomes aware that her discourse is not entirely matched by activity. She is willing to act, along with her son and about fifteen of his friends 'if the money is there to support us'. As noted by Ilkhamov (2005: 304) in Uzbekistan,

> although one can not doubt the commitment to the public interest of the majority of NGOs, at the same time it cannot be denied that the overflow of funds has created a sort of market of jobs and charity offers, a market driven more by the logic of supply and demand than the needs of civil society.

The outcome of such an approach has been a series of donor-organized NGOs (or, inevitably, DONGOs).[7]

In the meantime, she is the only one in the NGO who is actually working. As a consultant working under the auspices of her organization, she gives training sessions on HIV in certain local institutions. The number of workshops she does each year is limited, as she says: 'I can't do any more without a larger budget'. While Boda may be the only local NGO in the region to be truly active in the response to HIV prior to the arrival of IDO, it operates at a tiny scale and in a potentially explosive environment (i.e., the mutual hatred between Tatiana and Eldar).

The final type of group contacted by the IDO team at this stage is what they call 'nascent' NGOs. These are groups of friends with no formal organization or legal status, such as addict support groups and gay groups who exist in the face of both legal and social homophobia. At this stage, it must be remembered, HIV has not yet erupted in the region, and the determinant factors of the potential epidemic are not yet known. Nonetheless, available indicators suggest to Beth, Anna, Igor and their colleagues that the region's rising prevalence of injecting drug use could be behind a number of cases of infection. 'Are there local NGOs providing any assistance to addicts in the region?' asks the team working in the field. 'If so, we will help them develop some HIV prevention activities for injecting drug users, and thus potentially shield them from the epidemic.' What they find is that there are no NGOs working with addicts in the post-Soviet Caucasus and Central Asia at this time.

There is a reason for this. The USSR both criminalized and medicalized drug use through its state 'detoxification centres'. And this has continued in the independent republics of the region. The Soviet influence remains visible in the repressive, psychiatric approach to drug use, and in its definition of drug use as a criminal offence. For example, Soviet law distinguishes between consumption and trafficking using two criteria: the quantities of drugs seized and the financial motivation (possession with or without intention to sell). Soviet law emphasizes imprisonment and duress to both deter and treat drug users. There is no tradition of health care approaches for drug users (Bisiou 2004: 33).

After the fall of the USSR, these 'detoxification centres' continued to practise the same methods, while at the same time their working conditions deteriorated and their funding was disrupted. Some people still become 'patients' voluntarily, but more often the police bring them in, charging them with 'consumption' of illicit drugs. In fact, it is the police who decide if a person is charged as a drug user and under what criteria. Just possessing a syringe can be considered proof of drug use in the eyes of the militia. Those unable to pay a bribe are either sent directly to prison or to a detoxification centre, which is often nothing more than a preliminary stop on the way to prison. The centres are run jointly by the Ministry of the Interior (the prison service) and the Ministry of Health, and are in reality detention centres. 'Care' is limited to enforced abstinence, some tranquillizers if the patient can afford them, and occasionally hypnosis. As police activity lets up, forced hospitalizations have become rare. Voluntary registration has fallen sharply, partly because services must now be paid for.

When IDO arrives in the region, these centres are almost empty, populated mostly by ageing, depressed personnel. The most active have quit, emigrated or changed fields. Those who still work there – doctors, paramedics and security staff – recognize that they have had no impact on drug use. The also know about the risk of HIV infection, and it worries them. Nonetheless, the majority are still convinced that it would be best to return to the Soviet model of control of individuals who are 'dangerous to society'. For this they need funding to bring their centres back to their former state (this is much the way Eldar and his colleagues think about the Soviet system for HIV control). A few are open to new ideas – why not try non-governmental approaches, parallel to or in competition with the existing centres?

Such is the case with a small group that has formed around Piotr, a doctor and toxicology specialist who is director of one of the large national centres for narcology (state institutions involving drugs and drug abuse reporting to Ministries of Health). This group is typical of 'nascent' NGOs: it wants to carry out HIV prevention among drug users differently from the repressive state institutions, whose dark secrets and public health limitations they know well. They have not yet made their move at the time of IDO's arrival, partly because of doubts about the country's legal system and partly because of a lack of resources. When IDO enters the picture, their main constraint is not knowing how to get started. We'll learn more about Piotr at the end of this chapter.

Searching for gay men

When the IDO team starts looking for nascent local NGOs to join in HIV prevention, they have in mind (in addition to the danger of an explosive epidemic among drug users) the experience of gay groups in the United States and Europe. As described in the previous chapter, these NGOs created an extraordinary social movement of advocacy, HIV prevention and accompaniment of people living with the virus.[8] The IDO team looks for such groups to try to convince them to create their own anti-AIDS NGOs, and is prepared to help them do it. But they find that either such groups do not exist or face huge challenges to getting organized, again for reasons related to the post-Soviet context. The situation is difficult for the *goluboi*, as they call themselves. While their legal situation varies from one country to another, in most of the region even the suspicion of homosexuality can bring imprisonment.

Up until the 1980s in the Soviet Union, homosexuals were considered 'deviants' or 'sick' people who needed to be either punished or treated. It had not always been so: the USSR had a brief period during which homosexuality was decriminalized, in contrast to the vast majority of countries at the time. But in 1934 'sodomy' (*muzhelozhstvo*) became a crime punishable by five years in prison under Article 121 of Stalin's Criminal Code. Described at the time by Nikolai Krilenko, the People's Commissioner in charge of Justice, as a sign of the bourgeoisie's moral decadence and an anti-proletarian act, homosexuality came to be associated with the old order and was considered 'anti-revolutionary' (Kon 1995). Exact figures as to how many victims were punished pursuant to Article 121 are unknown, the archives currently being closed (De Jong 1982). Even if the archives are one day made public, making sense of the statistics will be complicated by the fact that many Soviet homosexuals were convicted of charges not covered by Article 121 such as 'hooliganism', or being a 'class enemy' (Gessen 1994; Kon 1995). The law was a powerful tool of repression, using homosexuality (or the suspicion of homosexuality) to prosecute and condemn a number of dissidents, or to keep a number of people detained in camps. Those condemned under this law were subject to violence and persecution by their co-detainees. While imprisonment was an extreme expression of homophobia, the social environment also served to marginalize and exclude homosexuals, forcing them into clandestine encounters and into meeting places that were quickly known to the authorities, in constant fear of being 'outed', with all the consequences that entailed.

Prejudice against homosexuals was reinforced by the arrival of the epidemic once the principle modes of transmission were well known. In 1985, Nikolai Burgasov, the Deputy Minister of Health, declared that 'any great increase in HIV/AIDS infection rates is impossible in the Soviet Union, as homosexuality is severely punished by our Criminal Law Code' (Burgasov 1986). Soviet anti-AIDS measures at the beginning of the 1990s, by virtue of their vague language, permitted homosexuals to be prosecuted and forced to have blood tests (Kon and Riordan 1993). Such veiled repression, social ostracism and the lack of anonymity for serological tests all constituted a brake on voluntary testing. Soviet men who had sex with other men had every reason to distrust testing services, knowing that if they went there they would be met with hostility, lack of confidentiality and stigmatization. Those who tested positive were reluctant to divulge their sexual orientation. The low number of positive diagnoses at the time suggests that the presence of HIV in the male homosexual population was underestimated (Mikkelsen 1996).

In such a context, it was almost impossible to create associations to defend minority rights, as in the West. A few exceptions existed in the European portion of the USSR, though not in the Caucasus or Central Asia. In 1984, for example, about thirty young people in Leningrad created an informal gay and lesbian group led by Aleksandr Zaremba. They named their group the 'Gay Laboratory'. Working with a Finnish group, they were able to send information to the West about the unenviable status of gays in the USSR, and asked to receive information about the emerging HIV epidemic. Placed under surveillance by the KGB and victimized by threats and repression (Zaremba was put in prison), some emigrated while others retreated into silence, re-surfacing only in the final years of *glasnost* (Kon 1995; Schluter 2002). In the meantime, *glasnost* gave rise to demands for liberalization of the legal framework around homosexuality. While this came mainly through pressure by groups at the fringes of mainstream opinion, their demands for abrogation of the principal article of the 1934 law (Article 121) found a degree of support in the written press, where a timid debate on the subject began, often linking homosexuality with bolshevism, Zionism and democracy. For the first time in the Soviet Union, homosexuality was the subject of a public debate, discussed not only in journalistic articles, but also in letters from homosexuals and their relatives. Many readers discovered for the first time the extent to which homosexuals were discriminated against, the police brutality they faced, the solitude they experienced and the rejection they had to deal with (Kon 1995). While the debate was launched by journals in favour of fighting homophobia, the subject was also discussed in the more conservative press. The latter, homophobic for the most part, reflected the views of the Soviet majority.

Taking advantage of the new atmosphere, a hitherto inconceivable study was carried out by the Soviet Centre for Study of the Public Opinion, which investigated attitudes towards homosexuality among Soviet citizens in different republics. The results spoke for themselves. Homophobia was prevalent throughout the Soviet Union. Of those interviewed, 64.4 per cent showed strong hostility towards homosexuals. When asked what should be done with homosexuals, 33.7 per cent stated that they should be killed, or, to use a Stalinist term, 'liquidated' and 30.7 per cent said they should be 'isolated from the rest of society' (Schluter 2002).

It was only at the very end of the Soviet regime that the first gay movement was born in Russia: the Association of Sexual Minorities. This described itself as 'an association for the defence of human rights, with the objective of obtaining complete equality between people of different sexual orientations' (Kon 1995). Its first media campaign demanded abrogation of Article 121, a change of the authorities' 'attitude to sexual minorities, and a declaration of amnesty for people imprisoned because of their sexual orientation'. The Association split due to internal conflicts and was replaced by the more local Moscow Union of Lesbians and Homosexuals. The legal situation for sexual minorities improved considerably in some republics of the former USSR, as countries such as Ukraine, Estonia, Lithuania and Moldova rapidly repealed Article 121 and decriminalized homosexuality. Under Western pressure, the Russian president Boris Yeltsin followed suit in 1993. The gay movement grew simultaneously in Russia and the republics closer to Europe (Ukraine and the Baltic states), with organizations publishing magazines such as *Risk*, *1/10*, *Impulse* and *SPID-info*.

The situation was very different in the Caucasus and Central Asia, where Article 121 remained in force (except in Armenia) and no specifically gay organizations existed. Discrimination against homosexuals remained strong and no officially sanctioned organization (NGO or other) represented them or even contemplated doing so. Little data on homosexual behaviour was available, but such research as existed (particularly Flowers 1991; Kalinin 1990; Oostvogels 1997; Oostvogels and Mikkelsen 1998) showed that many of those who identified themselves as homosexual were married, that condoms were rarely used and that gays and lesbians were still victims of humiliation and violence. Some received death threats and, to the visible indifference of the police, some of these were carried out.

This is the context in which the IDO team hopes to support gay groups. Their aim is to assist the growth of anything that might eventually create local NGOs interested in fighting HIV, and they begin their search for gay groups that might do so. The following scene is illustrative of dozens of others. On a Sunday morning in summer, Mike and I are invited to have coffee at the home of Anton, who is part of a group of young gays. We enter a turn-of-the-century building that would have looked at home in Haussmann's Paris, though grubby from overcrowding. We climb several staircases, and ring the doorbell. Silence, then some muffled footsteps. Behind the door, cloth pads slide over the parquet floor; and the door is opened by a little *babushka* of at least 80, her face lined by life, a flowered scarf around her head. There is a strong smell of cabbage as we walk down a long corridor, and she ushers us into a room on the left. The walls are covered in photos cut out of Western magazines showing handsome, muscled young men wearing very little. Our hostess returns carrying a platter, and we drink tea. She is a neighbour of Anton, and watched him grow up. Anton shares the collective apartment with her and four other families. He now has his own room, the one in which we find ourselves. 'He's coming', she says, excusing him affectionately, 'he went to a party last night, you understand ...' To help us pass the time, she tells the story of Anton as a child. In the middle of her story, Anton arrives with his friends. He closes the door, and although we can hear neighbours and their children getting up around us, it is as if the room has become separate from the rest of the flat. Anton and Yuri keep their voices low as they tell us about the difficult lives of homosexuals in the former USSR – one of the neighbours is a homophobe ...

Governments in the region do not always approve of IDO's interest in gay groups. I witnessed two types of reaction. The following illustrates the first, one of threats and intimidation. One day in 1995, Mike is threatened with expulsion by a government official for 'illegal activities'. Mike is an American citizen and a founder of one of the first NGOs doing HIV prevention in a Latin American country. In pure Soviet style, the official first speaks to me (a third party) to test the waters. Then, during one of Mike's absences, the official tells Beth about the government's displeasure and the reasons for expulsion: Mike has apparently sympathized with 'illegal groups' and thus 'threatens the security of the country'. Anna replies that in her opinion, IDO would counter-threaten a full range of diplomatic reprisals against the official if Mike were harassed. The threat is quickly withdrawn.

It should not be assumed that the hostility in official circles against permitting gay activist groups is in any way systematic. Some officials adopt a more flexible attitude, whether to maintain good relations with IDO or because they are actually coming to understand the invaluable role of gay activists in the global response to HIV/AIDS. Thus, in another country from the one in which Mike was threatened, it is the authorities themselves who try to include gay leaders in the national response. As Vladimir, the country's state secretary for AIDS, explains to the IDO team, 'we are in contact with a group of homosexuals, although it's illegal here and we don't approve of their behaviour. We believe they can play an important role in prevention, so we feel obliged to work with them. At least, that's what we'd like to do ... But they can't declare themselves openly as an organization, given that homosexuality is illegal ... We can't work directly with them for the moment, and even if it were possible, we aren't sure how we'd actually do it.'

It is Vladimir who arranges the first meeting between Alexey and the IDO team. Alexey is about 20. With a handful of friends, he has decided to spread awareness 'about the dangers of the AIDS epidemic' in general, but especially in his own country, where the phenomenon is largely unknown or denied by the authorities, and where – as in other post-Soviet societies – the weight of homophobia is heavy. Such information as Alexey and his friends have been able to obtain comes from foreign television programmes – from Turkey, the Middle East, Asia and so on. His first step was to get in touch with the government service 'in charge of fighting the epidemic', and it is there he met Vladimir, to whom he explained – warily – that he was looking for information. In confidence, he then stated his real objective: to raise awareness among the country's homosexuals. But what should he do? The IDO team learned about Alexey and asked to meet this small group to provide them with advice and support.

At the beginning of the meeting Alexey is tense and guarded, but he relaxes little by little as he explains the difficulties he faces, such as the lack of a publicly visible organization specifically for gays and the scarcity of places for them to meet in town. The 1934 law has not been used recently, but the threat is always there. At all costs they must avoid being identified by the police, because if charged with a contravention of the law, they risk repeated harassment and interrogations. When Anna asks him about the objective of creating an NGO, Alexey replies, 'What do you mean, an NGO?' Yes, 'they want to create a group. More and more people are getting sexually transmitted infections, particularly gays. We need money to provide treatment, and to educate them, because the country is no longer isolated from the rest of the world and HIV will be here sooner or later. But how do we proceed if it's illegal? They'll never authorize an overtly homosexual organization.'

Mike and Anna advise him to establish an NGO whose public goal would be preventing HIV/AIDS among young people, thus avoiding the term homosexuality and possible prosecution. They explain that this strategy has been used by many gay groups in other countries where discrimination was a significant problem. It has even helped groups to become prominent in the struggle to recognize the rights of sexual minorities. Alexey says this way of working interests him a lot, but that he and his friends feel isolated and uninformed about what such groups are doing in other countries, and they have no way of contacting them.

Negotiating in order to help

Far from undermining the bases of the institutional ideology being constructed by IDO, the near-absence of local NGOs working against AIDS, the diversity of the groups they are trying to enlist in the prevention effort, and the Soviet legacy in the areas of sexuality, contraception, and repression of drug use and homosexuality – all of these incite the IDO team to accelerate their activities in the Caucasus and Central Asia.

This stage, the longest and most visible one, sees their advocacy in favour of local NGOs at its height, and begins the implementation of an actual strategy of technical and material assistance. As we will see, after years of contact with each other, the government officials and local NGO members on one hand, and the IDO team members on the other, are beginning to really understand each other's ideas and practices. Having learned their respective points of reference, they have strengthened their own positions and advanced in their thinking, and are sometimes even able to joke about their own concepts and practices as well as those of other people.

The conditionality of aid

The IDO team are now ready to negotiate the conditions under which their aid is offered.[9] Long discussions begin between the agency and the governments of the region. John, the head of IDO, imposes some specific conditions for the release of funds. In his words, 'the government representatives were surprised that we didn't accept their proposals immediately. Some development agencies aren't that rigorous. HIV prevention, which no other international agency is currently promoting in the region, is a 'niche' activity for agencies to invest in because the epidemic is, unfortunately, going to explode and requests for assistance are going to increase. We could have put IDO's name on this niche without giving serious thought to what ought to be done ... That's how it often works in the development business, unfortunately. But we preferred to hang tough. Before we provided any aid, we insisted that governments abandon mass testing and contact tracing, and that they promote civil society initiatives.'

IDO undertakes these negotiations because it needs the approval of the governments in order to implement large-scale projects for the non-governmental sector. One might well ask why these governments are willing to sign agreements that will benefit local NGOs, which at this point are still disdained by the authorities. The reason is IDO's policy of conditionality. As we have seen in earlier chapters, these governments are asking for IDO's help because they no longer have the financial means to combat the epidemic. In line with the Soviet approach to the virus which they have not so far questioned, their priority request is for testing materiel and for assistance in producing and disseminating prevention messages. IDO does not accept the first of these requests because, at that time, the World Health Organization considers the region's testing resources to be sufficient, and 'if the governments wish to carry out mass testing, they should finance it themselves. We [the development agencies] do not wish to encourage such practices.' In contrast, government requests in the fields of information, education and communication are accepted.

The assistance given to governments is therefore conditional on their engagement in the 'flowering of civil society' (to use IDO's phrase) as part of their response to HIV. This policy of tit-for-tat plays out in the form of bargaining between John, Beth, Igor, Anna and their colleagues, and government actors like Eldar and Vladimir. For example, one of the typical demands is for reform of legislation on associations: all who apply should be able to enjoy official status, should not be harassed or pressured, and their activities should be free from political control. People are indeed regularly facing administrative barriers to the registration of NGOs. In addition, mandatory re-registration is often requested by governments of the region with the aim 'to filter out those undesirable, i.e., too independent' (Ilkhamov 2005: 301). At the same time, IDO is negotiating the apportioning of aid budgets. Assistance is refused if the government authorities request materiel for mass testing, as the agency makes explicit its disapproval of the practice. In the country where Eldar is state secretary for AIDS, for example, the IDO team states its position to the government as follows: 'If at least 50 per cent of our technical and financial assistance is not used to support local NGOs – like Boda and other less specialized agencies such as women's groups, reproductive health NGOs, those working on human rights, NGOs composed of young people or students or journalists, etc. – we will not provide funding.'

It is striking that the goal of this aid-related conditionality has remained to ensure a governmental environment that is favourable to the 'emergence and strengthening of civil society'. Such a strategy of demands and negotiations with governments is not the approach taken by all international agencies working in the former Soviet republics. Some reveal themselves to be less vigilant regarding local government practices, even if they are providing larger sums than IDO.

Financial assistance

The strategy of conditionality is reflected in the financing provided to information and HIV prevention activities of local NGOs. Contrary to what one might expect, IDO's financial assistance is not large compared to that of other agencies, which at this time are also beginning to finance local NGOs. NGOs only receive a few thousand pounds from IDO for their anti-HIV activities. Compared to local salaries, these sums seem substantial. But this is relative because IDO places ceilings on the proportion of its budgets that can be used to finance personnel costs, ceilings which can be only be raised for longer-term projects, normally for one to two years. Though small, the budgets cover a large number of NGOs. These fall into two types. The first are existing NGOs that are not yet active in HIV prevention but wish to be. The second, like Boda and, several years later, Sisao, are local NGOs whose main goal is to fight HIV/AIDS.

To help decide which projects to finance in each country, IDO has set up a selection system which is as transparent as possible. This is both to avoid the influence of pressure from any source, and to make it impossible for a limited group of well-informed actors – particularly those close to powerful political circles – to become the only candidates for financing. Beth, Igor and their colleagues publish their requests for proposals in the local press in order to reach the greatest number of people. They also bring together local civil society actors (professional associations of journalists and doctors, human rights groups), government specialists and foreigners involved in development work in the region (members of other international agencies) to create a temporary and independent authority charged with selecting projects from the proposals received. Certainly, this effectively limits the possibility of pressure or the corruption which is so widespread in the post-Soviet context. The Soviet legacy is still strong: IDO receives frequent proposals from public or private actors wearing their new NGO 'clothes', who are merely trying to obtain financing for activities which pay little heed to IDO's oft-repeated principles of good governance and effective HIV/AIDS work. Yet it should be emphasized that the majority of proposals from local NGOs are accepted. The rare ones that are rejected have not provided any details about their proposed activities, nor the budgets needed to carry them out. Practically all proposals receive financial support. We will analyse this phenomenon below, finding that during the first years of IDO's work with and through local NGOs, it is the strengthening of civil society that is the agency's main focus, rather than the nature and content of the proposed prevention activities.

'Technical' assistance

Parallel to the conditionality of aid described above, and material support for existing or emerging local NGOs, the agency pursues its advocacy for local NGOs with a large number of its partners under the guise of 'technical assistance'. It does this in the same way as it did at the beginning of its presence in the region, through public meetings and encounters with informal groups, with the aim of disseminating the ideas that underpin its institutional ideology. It also offers training sessions on HIV/AIDS and the techniques developed by NGOs in other parts of the world to fight the epidemic. These aim to 'build capacity' among existing or nascent NGOs, giving them the means to undertake effective HIV prevention activities.

As a volunteer in a rural women's group asks Beth, 'What exactly do you mean by *capacity building*?' A typical response is the following: 'NGOs can't be expected, in this desperate economic climate, to maintain their commitment without adequate human and financial resources. They have to be assisted, and it is this assistance that we call capacity building. For example, NGOs need training in designing and implementing anti-HIV activities, managing programmes, planning, raising funds, etc. It's a long process, during which the trainees transmit their skills to others in order to ensure the continuity and sustainability of their programmes.'

The training sessions bring together all the actors we have described earlier: members of local NGOs, informal groups, 'common' citizens, health professionals and government interlocutors – in other words, everyone with a personal or professional stake in the epidemic. The dates of these training sessions are announced in the press to reach as wide an audience as possible. It is therefore a period rich in encounters and exchange of ideas among people who otherwise have little opportunity to air and debate their different points of view. The sessions work according to a schema developed in other countries, both in the West and elsewhere. The facilitators begin by presenting the basic information about the virus itself and about its modes of transmission. Next come discussions of the different sexual practices that increase the risk of infection and the ways individuals can protect themselves. The third part is devoted to the experiences of NGOs active in HIV/AIDS in other parts of the world. The themes discussed range from the design and implementation of prevention activities to financial and personnel management issues such as how to handle volunteers. Fourth, IDO team members help the participants to do their own 'situation analyses' (to use IDO's terminology), describing what they do or could do, their strengths and weaknesses, and so on. Fifth, mini-sessions for 'strategic planning' are organized, in which the facilitators help participants to create, critique and improve 'business plans'. At this stage, and beyond the issue of HIV/AIDS, these training sessions help the participant develop skills in such areas as project management, organizational development, fundraising and information technology, as do other types of training offered to local NGOs members by international organizations in the region (Stevens 2005). The final stage is devoted to exploring the different types of activity that NGOs could carry out: psychological support before and after HIV testing, opening a telephone 'hotline' for counselling and informing people, methods of raising awareness in public places, fighting legal discrimination and so on.[10]

Study tours to other countries

Another part of technical assistance is foreign study tours, which IDO organizes for groups of local actors, both governmental and non-governmental. The visit of a group from Central Asia to Amsterdam in 1998 is a good example. The delegates have been chosen by the IDO team to be as representative as possible, with members of local NGOs already doing or intending to start HIV/AIDS activities, and government officials who have dealings with local NGOs in their country. It is an opportunity for them to see in action the ideas they have been debating with the IDO team. Amsterdam has been chosen for the vigour of its NGOs and their involvement in municipal public health. The tour objective is to meet the actors in a city where civil society, and particularly NGOs, are key elements in the response to HIV/AIDS. The Netherlands are known for the strength of their voluntary associations, whether organized according to group identity or to shared risk factors.

Before the trip, meetings are organized in Amsterdam with some twenty NGOs and government institutions representing the range of actors working against HIV/AIDS in the city. The aim is to ensure that the Central

Asian visitors' view of the situation in Amsterdam will be as representative as possible, and that they will see the extent to which the ideas being proposed to them exist in the 'real world'. These visits to institutions or associations providing support to people living with HIV/AIDS, groups of drug users, police in red light districts, prostitutes' NGOs, staff of the bus that distributes methadone and so on, prove to be like trips to other planets. The three visits that provide the strongest impressions are described below.

The first of these is to an 'association of people living with HIV/AIDS, open to all HIV-positive individuals and their friends and family', as one of its members describes it. The association is divided into sections representing different categories of members: HIV-positive women, users and ex-users of drugs, prisoners and so on. It has three goals: information, promoting the interests of people living with HIV/AIDS, and providing support and mutual assistance. 'Since 1990', they say, 'we have brought together all the information that might help HIV-positive people and anyone who is looking for information on the virus. You can get it from our office but also from the Internet, from our bi-monthly newsletter, and in the evening events that we regularly organize in cafés around the country . . . We don't prescribe anything, but access to information can help people make personal decisions, or can motivate them.'

Mutual assistance includes a range of activities, from support for people who can no longer look after themselves alone, to a hotline, potluck dinners and organizing parties and get-togethers in cafés.

The Central Asians learn that the NGO is also very active in fighting discrimination against HIV-positive people by employers, insurance companies and in areas such as housing and travel. The work covers both collective rights and individual cases of people needing help. A member continues: 'The association makes sure the government and the nation's institutions respect the rights of people living with HIV/AIDS. We keep tabs on conditions in hospitals and denounce practices that don't meet government commitments. We do the same with insurance companies and employers who don't respect HIV-positive people's human rights. It may seem innocuous, but actually our actions have a long reach – these institutions know they are being watched and risk lawsuits or media campaigns against them, so they think twice about messing with us . . . The important thing is for society to understand that people living with HIV/AIDS are organized and ready to react. Prejudice is never far away when you're dealing with this epidemic.'

Fighting prejudice is precisely the reason why about thirty members of the organization invite us to share lunch with them. This provokes strong emotion from the Central Asians, the large majority of whom have never knowingly crossed paths with an HIV-positive individual (remember that prevalence in their part of the world is still extremely low in 1998) – which is why the Dutch have extended this invitation. We are all aware of this event's political implications, particularly for the government representatives who, in the post-Soviet era, still are not publicly associated with HIV-positive people. But this is also the case for some of the NGO actors: Igor cannot take the intimacy of the event, and quietly goes out to the street. His compatriots do not criticize him, and nothing is said about his leaving.

'He's afraid of getting infected', whispers Lena. 'He'll change. It was important that we came to this lunch, including the most conservative of us. It shows that we are all beginning to change. Even me, and I think I was one of the most open-minded. Today I've learned that I still haven't faced the most important issue. We are still protected from the epidemic in our region. It allows people to pass the buck, even though in reality we can no longer afford to do so.'

The impression made on the visitors is similar at their meeting with a gay and lesbian NGO active in HIV prevention, whose prevention and health education unit hosts the meeting. Even before the meeting starts, the visitors are amazed by the NGO's offices. 'You'd think you were in the headquarters of IBM', Vladimir whispers to me as we go through the entrance. It is an ultra-modern building, spacious and superbly equipped with computers, lots of meeting rooms and so on, far beyond anything in even the best-funded post-Soviet ministries of health. The Central Asians stare open-mouthed at the explicit posters on the walls, trying to square the (for them) 'anti-social' images with the visible respectability of the NGO's office and members. Vladimir leans over to me and quietly asks, 'They're gay? All of them? But they seem normal!'

Later on he asks the NGO members, 'How many homosexuals are there in Amsterdam?' Julian, a member of the prevention unit, replies, 'About 45,000'. The Central Asians exchange looks, astounded by the figure. Julian guesses the next question and adds, 'Out of 700,000'. Vladimir nods, both interested and uncomfortable, and asks, 'And how many are infected?' Julian says, 'Only 4 per cent to 7 per cent are seropositive. Because of the work of NGOs like ours, prevention seems to work very well in Amsterdam among gay men.' The Central Asians learn about the organization's mini-projects in public parks, saunas, discotheques and 'backrooms'. They find the most striking activities to be the 'guerrilla sex parties' that are regularly organized. 'These are shows that we put on in gay bars and night clubs', says Julian, 'with prevention workers dressed in guerrilla uniforms'. As Julian describes them, an invitation poster is passed around the table: men in black and red leather G-strings – 'Very hot shows, and really effective for delivering prevention messages and changing certain types of behaviour', comments one of our Dutch hosts. Mirna, a member of a Central Asian NGO, cannot believe it: 'And you're supported by the government?' Julian replies in the affirmative: 'The authorities, both national and municipal, support us [a calculated pause] and finance us'.

The third outstanding visit for the Central Asians is to an NGO created in 1909 to fight alcoholism, which now works with drug users. Robert, one of its members, tells us that there are about five or six thousand in the city, of whom between 50 per cent and 60 per cent inject their drugs.[11] 'We offer two alternatives: detoxification treatment, or support in reducing or stabilizing their consumption.' This double strategy, particularly the latter, has kept HIV prevalence among the city's drug users at low levels (about 2 per cent at time of writing, versus 9 per cent in 1989). 'Actually, as far as we can see, the second alternative gives better results in terms of individuals' health', says Robert. 'It's best to accept other people's behaviour, whatever it is, and help them live better. Living better means they also protect the other people in their lives. For that, you need to help them avoid certain risk factors. For example, the high cost of drugs results in practices – like prostitution, but that's not the only one – that can put them in danger.'

Mirna asks, 'But how do you do that?' Robert answers, 'By procuring substitute drugs for them, for example. You've visited the methadone bus, haven't you?' They have, that very morning. 'It's possible that some of them might eventually receive their drugs for free', adds Robert. 'The municipality is thinking about it. That way, they wouldn't be driven to situations that put them at risk of HIV infection simply because they needed money to buy drugs.'

'They've gone crazy', comments Vladimir, aside. The Dutch are explaining their position on testing. 'Until recently we didn't recommend testing to drug users who came to us, because treatment wasn't affordable. In the absence of treatment, we considered the essential objective to be helping the individuals to protect themselves and the people in their lives, whether they were HIV-positive or not. But now we counsel them to get tested so that they can get treatment as soon as possible if they need it.'

Robert notes that this position is not shared by all of the community actors in Amsterdam, and explains the different arguments. The Central Asians are amazed, especially by the long history and professionalism of the organization, which has been praised by all of the local actors in Amsterdam.

In Holland the delegates are experiencing things they have been hearing about from the IDO team for the past three years. Though aware that Amsterdam provides only one possible version of the ideas advocated by the agency, the visit has been very important for them. For the first time, they have seen the political force and media clout that groups of people living with HIV/AIDS can have. This is not new to them because of their discussions with the IDO, but, as they say one night in their hotel, 'it's as if it is only today that it becomes real'.

The hotel is our home during the visit. After days spent with the Dutch NGOs and their partners, we always get together in one or another of our rooms to have dinner. The price of one lunch in a restaurant has dissuaded them from going out for meals. They've decided that the money IDO gives them to cover the costs of their trip would be more useful to take home to their families. Cheese and sausages, tea, Soviet-built electric kettles for travellers, and a variety of alcohol emerge from their suitcases. The conviviality of Central Asian evenings is reproduced alongside an Amsterdam canal. Between songs, the debates are reopened. One day, someone whispers to me, 'You know, the existence of this kind of thing used to seem impossible. Groups of friends becoming professional institutions; marginals who would have ended up in prison a few years ago becoming the guardians of the rest of the population's health; private enterprise that defends the public good ... From now on, the inconceivable reigns!'

Glass of vodka in hand, another says, 'And to actually shake hands with the inconceivable, if only its Dutch version, that's really something!'

A new NGO

Advocacy, conditionality, funding, technical assistance and transfer of knowledge: these different facets of the agency's work can be illustrated by the assistance given to the group that has formed around Piotr, the doctor we have already met who specializes in working with addicts.

As we have seen, during the third phase of construction of IDO's institutional ideology, the team members get in touch with both professionals from the state 'detoxification centres' and injecting drug users in hopes of finding potential partners. What they find is an approach to treatment for addiction that was essentially coercive and institutional, and a total absence of drug users' NGOs due to stigmatization, discrimination and criminalization of drug consumption. They also learn that some professionals from the centres (the only institutions working in this field at the time) are interested in what the IDO had to say because – facing the gradual deterioration of their working conditions and conscious of the limited usefulness of their approach to addicts – they are looking for new tools to do their work. After numerous discussions with Beth, Anna and their colleagues, Piotr leaves his state centre and decides to create the NGO Narco with the help of former colleagues, patients (both current and former addicts) and groups of students. Narco's goal is to help injecting drug users protect themselves from HIV. Piotr realizes – in fact, is amazed by – IDO's willingness to condition its support to the government on benefits to someone as powerless as himself and his group. At the same time, having grown up in the Soviet system, he is realistic about the need to assure ministry officials that he will cooperate with them and use his NGO status in an unthreatening way. He is unambitious but knows how the game is played. While he will acknowledge the failings and opportunism of the state officials and the new crop of non-profit entrepreneurs, he does not judge them harshly and in fact seldom comments on their motivations.

Lacking government support, the creation of the NGO is not easy. The state secretary for AIDS is Eldar who, as we have seen, tries to prevent any non-governmental initiative that is not under his control (an example is his feud with Boda, Tatiana's NGO). It is in part due to John, the local head of IDO, and his team that Narco is finally registered legally. John is obliged to use the conditionality of assistance to put pressure on the government. He also insists that HIV prevention activities among addicts be permitted in the country, along with reviewing the heavy-handed policy of criminalizing drug use. Even with the pressure of conditionality from IDO, it takes over a year for the Ministry of the Interior to accept from Piotr the documents necessary for registration.

From the moment Narco officially exists, the IDO actors provide it with technical and material support.[12] To familiarize it with the experience of other local NGOs working in the same field, they invite its members, along with any other interested organizations, to participate in a training session. They also invite an experienced member of a Baltic NGO to be part of the training. A former Soviet official, he is chosen for his knowledge of addicts' lives in the region and of working conditions in the detoxification centres, and the experience he has developed over several years in an NGO whose objectives are similar to the ones adopted by Narco. The Baltic countries, due to their proximity to Western Europe, have benefited since the beginning of the decade from massive amounts of international aid, and are well ahead of the Caucasus and Central Asia in this field. His participation in training Narco members will be followed by the latter's visit to the Baltic, organized and funded by IDO along the same lines as the Amsterdam study tour.

IDO adds technical assistance to its material support. Narco is provided with funding to develop risk reduction activities among addicts in the country's capital and then in the major cities. These include attacking social stigma against drug users, setting up needle and syringe exchanges, and distributing condoms and information about the epidemic. The NGO's independence is a source of constant problems with the authorities, particularly Eldar, who regularly tries to block supplies of needles and syringes or sends the police to the places where meetings and prevention activities are carried out. After a few years, however, Piotr manages to organize a drop-in centre for addicts, modelled on numerous examples in Europe and America. Situated on the ground floor of an apartment building and operated by the NGO, the centre provides psychological, medical and legal help to addicts, a needle and syringe exchange (old ones for new ones), condoms and information on HIV prevention. Services are anonymous and free, and there is also a telephone hotline.

Narco members dream of eventually providing substitution treatment such as methadone. For the moment, however, this is impossible due to resistance from the ministries of Health and the Interior, who are stuck in the Soviet approach to fighting drug use.

4 White, red and grey

In this chapter, the fourth act of this ethnography, the IDO actors revisit the initial tools of this agency's institutional ideology, and a new interpretation of that ideology is born. This involves a sort of 'filtering' process, in which the actors filter information about their partners and the surrounding context into two basic colours which are heavily symbolic to them: white and red. The dichotomy may be nuanced by each individual actor, but the only real differences of opinion concern which of their local partners should be categorized as white or red, rather than with the categories themselves. The local partners are classified as white if they are seen to be going in the direction of the 'flowering of civil society' sought by the agency, and red if they seem to be resisting this flowering as a result of their Soviet legacy.

White attitudes and behaviours are taken to be evidence that the institutional ideology is well founded in its assumption that pent-up reformist or 'progressive' forces existed in the region prior to the agencies' arrival. As one can read in internal IDO documents, of which this is a typical example, 'for many decades, non-governmental activities were forbidden and repressed, and volunteerism had no place except in the mass organizations controlled by the state. Successive generations have known only this monolithic structure of control, in which independent initiatives were limited to the personal sphere. Today, a renaissance can be seen in the form of the NGO.'

Red attitudes are also taken to be supporting evidence that local resistance to this ideology had its source in the 'the crushing of civil society' by the Soviet system.

The following pages present a number of illustrations of what the IDO actors consider red or white in their partners' evolution. They are followed by examples of a third colour – grey – which provides a more nuanced explanation of the changing attitudes and behaviour of both the IDO members and their local partners.

White

Three local NGOs stand out for the IDO team as examples of the white tendency: an NGO working with drug users (Narco), a gay NGO (Sisao) and one working on prevention at a more general level (Boda). All three are seen as archetypal examples of the 'universal' model that the agency supports, combining a resemblance to Western models within the constraints inherited from the Soviet context. We will examine Sisao and Boda more closely here.

As we have seen earlier, when the team was in contact with some informal gay groups, Anna and Mike recommended that Alexey create an NGO with the official objective of fighting HIV/AIDS, for example among young people. This would allow him to circumvent the criminalization of homosexuality and pervasive homophobia that make specifically gay NGOs impossible. In 1997, Alexey and his friends officially create an organization with the stated aim of preventing HIV among young people, but with the understanding that the gay population is their particular interest. Sisao has about twenty founding members, all in their twenties, who are well aware that they – members of the liberal professions or university students, city dwellers from the nation's capital – are not representative of the country's gay population. That very non-representativeness is one of their motivating factors, they say, for they hope that their struggle for the rights of sexual minorities will be of benefit to others who are disadvantaged socially or geographically.

But this official existence as a fully fledged NGO requires another important step from IDO: to ensure the decriminalization of homosexuality. In the middle of the 1990s, the prohibition of homosexuality under Article 121 of the Soviet Criminal Code is still in force in the countries of Central Asia and the Caucasus, with the exception of Armenia. It provides the underlying basis for the national laws in each of the region's countries, which begin to introduce their own modifications over time. For this reason, John, one of the heads of IDO in the region, together with his team, brings pressure to bear on the governments using the conditionality of aid described earlier. This pressure has two objectives: first, to decriminalize homosexuality; second, to permit the legal registration of gay NGOs. In addition to lobbying, and with the aim of 'assisting' certain governments to move from talk to action by amending their laws, the IDO staff commission an American legal expert to analyse existing legislation – that is, the Soviet one – and advise on its revision.

As pressure is brought to bear, three of the five Central Asian republics decriminalize homosexuality. The first is Kazakhstan in 1997, followed by Kyrgyzstan and Tajikistan in 1998. However, although this change is a real breath of fresh air for homosexuals in Kazakhstan and Kyrgyzstan, in Tajikistan it is merely cosmetic, with repression in the form of prison sentences continuing as before. As for Uzbekistan and Turkmenistan, attempts to make aid conditional were not enough to convince the national governments. In Uzbekistan, Article 120 of the new penal code passed in 1995 provides for three-year prison terms in cases of sodomy. In Turkmenistan, a new penal code was passed in 1997, but it is not known if the article criminalizing homosexuality was removed in the final document signed by the president.

Once homosexuality is decriminalized in a given country, the IDO staff lobby the government to permit the registration of local gay NGOs. In one of the countries, Alexey and his friends apply to the Ministry of the Interior, without whose authorization no NGO can exist. IDO has provided them with information about HIV prevention work in other parts of the world, which Alexey and his friend Slava have used to support their application. Sisao is officially recognized in 1997. This step is important, because once registered, an NGO can receive international aid – financial, material, technical – without having to ask the government for authorization. During its first years, it is headed by a young woman who is a friend of the group; this provides discreet 'cover' that the group judges necessary. In reality, the leader is Slava, as Alexey has emigrated in the meantime. Like all the members, Slava is not paid for his work. He is a tall, highly intelligent young man, whose manner is both shy and calm. From his considerable height, he leans eagerly towards his interlocutors, enveloping them with a gentle enthusiasm that even hardline homophobes find impressive. Nonetheless, Sisao has difficulties with its first activities. As Slava says, 'We don't know how to do things, or where to start. For the moment, we don't even have a place to do our work.' The group has to work through the questions common to most new NGOs working against HIV/AIDS: how to find information on HIV, how to present prevention information, how to procure condoms and organize their distribution, how to learn about the lives and needs of homosexuals outside the large cities and create activities to reach them, how to find and train volunteers and protect them from 'burnout', how to find funding for their activities and so on.

To expose them to the experiences of NGOs in Europe, Asia, Latin America and Africa, IDO invites them (along with all other interested local NGOs) to participate in the type of training sessions and discussions described in the previous chapter. The agency team also helps them carry out qualitative field studies which provide them with insights into the behaviour of the country's homosexuals and bisexuals. Mirna is a key asset in this activity. As a psychologist involved in women's rights, particularly the rights of prostitutes, she is hired by IDO to help the Sisao volunteers carry out these studies, which provide the evidence on which their activities will be based. IDO soon adds material support to its technical assistance, and provides the funding both for condom distribution and to publish HIV/AIDS information adapted specifically for gay men in the country. IDO and other international agencies' funds also permit Sisao to open a telephone service for a few days a week, providing information and the opportunity for anonymous discussion of sexuality, HIV/AIDS and sexually transmitted diseases.

Sisao's activities develop further over the years, thanks to the dynamism of its members. It participates in radio broadcasts, does outreach in public parks, trains volunteers to carry on the work in other parts of the country, creates the capital's first specifically gay bar and – on the floor above – opens an office where the public can meet Sisao members and learn about the epidemic. The profits from sales of tickets to the discotheque also provide some financial independence, giving Slava and his colleagues a freedom of action that is rare among NGOs in the region. Though modest, these extra funds help Sisao survive the inevitable fluctuations in funding from donors, who are always happy to cite Sisao as an example of 'best practice' but are particularly unforthcoming when it comes to providing finance, for fear of provoking the rampant homophobia of many officials. Each of its projects requires a separate application for funds, and funding renewal is neither automatic nor free from delays, which can leave gaps of several months between approved budgets. The system and its problems are common to all international development agencies and well known to NGOs, who learn to assemble a 'war chest' or independent sources of funds to assure the continuity of projects caught between agency budgets.

This ability to cope is all the more admirable given that, even in the countries where the legislation has changed, discrimination against homosexuals remains extremely strong. This is exemplified by a study carried out in the capital of Kyrgyzstan in 1998 among 100 homosexual men. Over ninety denounce the homophobia that surrounds them. Out of respect for their families and fear of discrimination, contacts between men are reported as limited, confined to closed groups of friends, with extreme distrust of outsiders. The study finds that forty-seven respondents are married or in a stable relationship with a woman. Lacking secure venues to meet in, certain areas in the large cities are identified as places for homosexual encounters (*pleshka* in Russian slang). These are often sections of streets with a lot of pedestrian circulation, with a park or square, public toilets, and metro or bus stations (in Tashkent, for instance). Public bath houses (*banyas*) are frequently used, as are certain downtown cafés and restaurants. Private apartments and *dachas* (holiday homes) are also cited as meeting places. More recently, the Internet has provided a much-appreciated way to meet and communicate as it is considered safer than physical locations known to the authorities. The fact remains that many homosexuals in the region receive anonymous death threats, some of which are treated with absolute indifference by the forces of law and order. Many homosexuals have little idea of their rights, and in Kazakhstan, Kyrgyzstan and Tajikistan many do not know that homosexuality has been legalized – a fact that the forces of law and order, if they themselves are aware, refrain from telling them. The most violent forms of discrimination stem from harassment by police and militias, who frequently use the threat of prosecution (whether under Article 121 in countries where it remains in force, through other charges such as 'hooliganism' – much used in Soviet times – or by arrest for murders or thefts committed by others in the area) as an excuse for extreme violence, or to extort written confessions which can then be used to extract *bakshish*, or to denounce other people. If the homosexual resists, he or she can expect to be sent to prison, where other forms of violence await, including sexual violence.

As in earlier times, persecution can also be carried out at a political level. The case of Ruslan Sharipov is indicative. A homosexual Uzbek journalist who headed an association defending the liberty of the press, he was arrested in 2003 after publishing a series of articles denouncing human rights violations in Uzbekistan. He was accused of sodomy and paedophilia, and was forced to write his confession after torture and death threats. His lawyer, Surat Ikramov, was kidnapped and severely beaten by hooded men while on his way to a meeting to prepare Sharipov's defence. The trial ended with Ruslan Sharipov being sentenced to five and a half years in prison, a term reduced on appeal to four years. After having received considerable attention from groups such as Amnesty International, Human Rights Watch and Reporters without Borders, Shapirov managed to escape from prison in 2004 and was granted refugee status in the United States.

Merely belonging to an NGO working for the rights of homosexuals can be dangerous. Two examples are illustrative. At the end of the 1990s, a local NGO carried out a small-scale study on homosexuality. Shortly after, an extremely hostile article was published in a local newspaper containing information collected by the study during interviews, which should have remained confidential. As well as resulting in physical and verbal harassment of the individuals involved, the incident cost the NGO a great deal of credibility and reinforced homosexuals' distrust and fear of being identified as such. The second example is even more extreme. In 2002, three young homosexuals who had been volunteers for a time were arrested by police on suspicion of having murdered a man, himself homosexual. They were condemned to prison with sentences ranging from fourteen to fifteen years; neither the police nor the court would take their evidence into account, as it was judged inadmissible due to their sexual orientation. The prison sentences manifestly put the young men at high risk, given that the practice of male rape is well documented in the regions' prisons. One of the three has apparently contracted tuberculosis while in prison and is in poor health.

It is in this context that, in 2003, Sisao launches a new project which is directly linked to its founding aims: working for the legal protection of sexual minorities. A new, younger generation of volunteers, many of them students, is mounting a human rights-based attack on homophobia. Boris has replaced Slava as leader. Though tired out by years of volunteer work on top of a regular job, Slava is still an active member of the group.

Boris is about 40 and works hard to avoid schisms in the group. Many of the members are burned out by the frequent disruptions of international agency funding, which oblige Boris and his friends to work intensely among the volunteers to convince them that they have not been abandoned, and to spend a great deal of time searching for new sources of funding. They are also exhausted by the persistent homophobia in the region. Nonetheless, the IDO and other international agencies' teams have proposed that members of Sisao, who are now 'experts' after many years of work, facilitate training sessions among police officers, prison guards and the clergy, and thereby continue the advocacy work once assumed by the agency. The energy, perseverance and now the professionalism of the Sisao members – all unpaid volunteers operating in a homophobic environment – has gained the respect of everyone, including some government officials. They have been able to maintain their organization's material and moral independence, and to stay true to their goals. To borrow the words of Parker, Khan and Aggleton about prevention programmes by gay men's groups in other parts of the world, Sisao's actions are a 'testament to the perseverance and courage [of people] that have confronted ongoing stigma, discrimination and, in some cases, outright violence, yet which have persisted, often with impressive success, in the face of such difficult conditions' (Parker, Khan and Aggleton 1998: 341).

The NGO Boda is another white organization that has grown considerably due to IDO support over the years. Boda was the only NGO already active in the response to HIV/AIDS before IDO arrived on the scene, although its activities were limited to occasional training sessions focusing on the basics of HIV transmission, provided by Tatiana, the only active member of the organization at the time.

As seen in the previous chapter, certain former Soviet associations which had rebaptized themselves as NGOs hoped to continue working in the same way they had done up until 1991, and expected donors to provide them with a programme that they could implement. The IDO team tried to communicate their concept of civil society, and asked in vain for these NGOs to explain what they hoped to do in the response, to which the NGOs replied that they expected to be provided with a 'plan'. Frustrated by this dialogue of the deaf, the IDO team hope that Tatiana might be able to help these new NGOs to change their approach, and ask her to convince these local NGOs to join in the response to HIV/AIDS with their own prevention activities.

As the agency had hoped, Tatiana proves extremely active. Taking up the team's discourse, she manages over time to convince the rebaptized former Soviet institutions and associations to create prevention projects and submit them to IDO and other international agencies for financing. In doing so, she follows the strategy adopted by the team when they first arrived in the region, but concentrates on bringing former *apparatchiks* into the picture. Their NGOs tend to need detailed guidelines before they start to plan anything, and Tatiana responds perfectly to that need. She helps them to define their potential areas of competence in HIV/AIDS, and trains some of their volunteers.

While Tatiana's work 'demonstrates' the success of their approach, she also gives rise to a certain amount of unease among the IDO team. Some of her attitudes remind them uncomfortably of her arch-enemy, Eldar. When IDO proposes to hire her, she demands the same perquisites she had as state secretary for AIDS (the post Eldar now occupies), and even a contract stipulating that she will 'create and direct the country's sole association of anti-AIDS non-governmental organizations'. These demands are refused by the agency. Another source of unease: little by little, the IDO team realize that in her work on their behalf, Tatiana only provides assistance to local NGOs of her own choice and rejects those she says that 'she cannot supervise'.

Eventually, the team members begin to wonder about Boda, which Tatiana continues to head. Over the years, they have noticed that she has systematically refused to introduce them to the members of her NGO or show them its work. The following brief exchange is representative of the way Tatiana uses the IDO discourse to reinforce her own position.

TATIANA (*delivering a presentation that could have been taken straight from one of IDO's HIV prevention manuals*): 'The main activity of the NGO Boda is HIV education and prevention through peer educators recruited from relevant target groups and trained with these objectives in mind. This peer education is carried out primarily in school settings but also in the private sector, among those working in the sex industry, and among both intravenous drug users and men who have sex with men ...'

MIKE (*trying to bring her around to the actual makeup of her NGO*): 'How many active volunteers do you have?'

TATIANA (*thrown off her stride*): 'I am unable to tell you that because they do not wish to be identified.' (*Returning to where she had left off in her discourse*) 'Other activities concern the organization of various competitions for the development and production of HIV-related educational materials, such as contests for the best article, the best poster, the best advertisement ...'

ANNA (*trying to interrupt her gently*): 'Would it be possible to meet some of your NGO's members?'

TATIANA: 'You realize, of course, that they cannot be forced to meet you ... The best way is to work through me.'

ANNA: 'I'm not asking for their names. All I want is to accompany them as they go about their work, the way I normally do with other NGOs.'

TATIANA: 'You must understand that our work doesn't follow a set schedule. It depends on the needs expressed by the groups themselves according to their own agendas, their comparative advantages and weaknesses ...'

MIKE (*annoyed by her regurgitation of international HIV programme clichés*): 'Look, it's kind of difficult to get any hard information on what your NGO is actually doing!'

TATIANA (*a fixed smile on her face*): 'More activity would be visible if appropriate resources were available. The real issue is inadequate levels of funding.'

Seeing Tatiana's attitude and how little substance there is behind her trumpeting of links with grassroots clients and all the right 'communities' from gay men to commercial sex workers, one perfectly understands the team members' reservations about Boda's activities. Yet it is striking how quickly these shortcomings are forgotten, such is their desire to see in Tatiana and Boda the affirmation of their approach. We will return to this later on.

While the team members tend to use Sisao, Boda and Narco as their prize examples of the evolution of local NGOs, they are equally proud of certain government actors whom they consider to be 'white'. Vladimir, who is still his country's state secretary for AIDS, is a good example. His evolution was already seen in its beginning stages in previous chapters, particularly in the study tour to Amsterdam. The following conversation shows how far he has come. This time, Vladimir is no longer debating with the IDO team but with his Ministry of Health colleagues in a remote mountain province, who remain proponents of the Soviet-era ideas he espoused only a few years before.

It is winter, in a snowbound provincial town with its central square, its People's Palace, its post and telecommunications office, its market – all typical of so many cities in the region. Beyond the rows of Soviet-style apartments along the four main streets, the houses are made of wood and the roads are unpaved. There is no longer any lighting in the streets, nor heat or hot water in the people's homes. The local factories, which had depended on the Soviet economy, are closed; their immense, rusting hulks line the roads. Half of the working-age population is unemployed. Salaries of people still employed by the state are only paid infrequently, and monthly state pensions are barely enough to buy bread for two days. A few local businesses have sprung up but no NGOs. The main concern of the population is survival.

One day, a meeting is organized in the *oblast* administrative headquarters on the theme of 'health and social issues, particularly HIV/AIDS'. The meeting room resembles those of *oblast* committees across the former USSR: a 1960s-style amphitheatre with a plywood podium and orange curtains. The cold is glacial. Some of the hundred or so people in the audience wear heavy coats and fur hats covering their ears. Some are district and village officials who still occupy the posts they had in Soviet times, while others are common citizens interested in hearing the discussion. On the podium, Vladimir becomes worked up as he describes the epidemiological situation of STIs and HIV in the former Soviet countries:

VLADIMIR: 'The epidemic is going to take off. It's simply inevitable: look at the STI levels. And what are you doing about it?'

AN *OBLAST* PUBLIC HEALTH OFFICIAL: 'We organize annual propaganda meetings on AIDS. Our doctors facilitate meetings with *oblast* authorities, medical students . . .'

VLADIMIR: 'HIV is not just a medical problem! It's a social issue! Civil servants like you cannot deal with it on your own. You've been doing these Soviet-style meetings for ten years now – have they changed anything?' (*Silence in the room.*) 'HIV is transmitted by sexual activity, among other routes. Are we going to prevent people from making love? Even Stalin couldn't manage that ...' (*A few embarrassed laughs. Vladimir pushes on.*) 'Our mindsets have to change! The Berlin Wall has fallen. I know it's hard to bring down the walls in our minds. But we simply don't have any choice.'

A VILLAGE OFFICIAL: 'What needs to be done, in concrete terms? What are you doing in the capital?'

VLADIMIR: 'We use the mass media to disseminate information created by groups of young people, vulnerable people, NGOs and so on, which ensures it will be attractive to the public. We organize discussions with the police and prison staff about respecting the rights of people who are HIV-positive or who want to be tested. We work with NGOs, women's groups, and associations of drug users, and we help them organize prevention outreach ...'

A FACTORY WORKER: 'Young people are seeing so much these days, the old values make no sense to them. What are we to say to them when we aren't sure of anything ourselves?'

A DISTRICT OFFICIAL: 'All we know is that we aren't happy with any of this.'

VLADIMIR: 'We have to think about prevention, based on the actual situation in the country. Not the past situation, or an ideal one, but today's conditions. That's why groups of people mobilizing around new ideas are essential. Sexual activity and drug use need to be done in safety ... Addicts need help to work collectively against the injection practices that put them at risk. We help them to distribute free needles and syringes, and to organize needle exchanges among their own networks. In your own *oblast*, for example, the international agencies have donated thousands of condoms. They need to be promoted and used! If groups of young people ask for them, they should receive them in quantity! Forget about distributing them only in institutional and medical settings. Giving them out one by one in clinics, maybe that helps someone here and there. But that approach has achieved nothing over the years. We need to shift into higher gear and reach people through informal groups, through people who get involved because they're afraid for themselves or their children or their friends – their motivation doesn't matter! We need to get organized and use NGOs to put pressure on the state. And yes, we need to change the way we think.'

AN *OBLAST* OFFICIAL: 'There are some young women who are committing immoral practices. This ought to be punished.'

VLADIMIR: 'You need to understand the situation. It's because of the current economic conditions that some women turn to prostitution for a living. Instead of condemning it or closing our eyes and pretending it doesn't exist, there should be local campaigns to make sure the clients use condoms and that the women are protected. That's what I saw in Amsterdam. I was amazed. The prostitutes in that city don't have STIs, and levels of HIV infection are very low.'

THE OFFICIAL: 'That sort of thing never used to be authorized.'

VLADIMIR: 'I know, I'm over 60 and I remember. Is that the best way to make a living? Do we need to accept it? I don't know. But who can stop it now? The police? Are the police even paid here? It's a miracle if they are, and I'll bet they'd be the only ones.'

ANOTHER OFFICIAL: 'In Soviet times, AIDS would never have arrived in our country.'

VLADIMIR: 'But it did arrive. That is the actual situation. And it's a grave threat.'

AN ELDERLY MAN: 'I'm the rector of the *oblast* university. Last year twelve students were diagnosed with STIs. But they refused to say who they'd slept with! And they are protected by the new legislation. It's unacceptable! I need this information so I can take the appropriate measures! We need to organize compulsory testing – then we'd know who is infected.'

VLADIMIR: 'I would have liked to retain that in the national HIV control policy. Testing for everyone. But we couldn't, because that would have been against the agreements we've signed with the international agencies. All you can do is try to persuade people. Now, we simply have to accept this new reality and work with it. If we want to persuade people to protect themselves, we'll need to get civil society to take responsibility.'

ANOTHER LOCAL: 'Before, under the Soviet Union, when there was an epidemic in a city it would be quarantined – end of story. No one could enter or leave.'

VLADIMIR: 'I'm glad you brought that up. But our country has signed agreements with the international agencies, and while they help us they also set limits on what we can do.'

THE DISTRICT MEDICAL OFFICER: 'I proposed to the *oblast* authorities that everyone be tested and that a medical certificate be necessary for anyone to enter. But they refused my proposal.'

AN *OBLAST* OFFICIAL: 'We can't ask for a medical certificate from everyone who enters the country. But we ought to organize testing in the sanatoriums, holiday centres, schools and other places like that.'

VLADIMIR: 'In any case, it would cost too much to test everyone, and we haven't the resources. So we need to adapt to the actual conditions and do prevention through other channels, particularly through NGOs.'

A LOCAL (*struggling to summarize*): 'Okay. The new policy says we can't force people. We can't convince them by argument. Therefore, they can't be controlled any more ... So what can we do?'

THE *OBLAST* PUBLIC HEALTH CHIEF (*banging his fist on the podium in front of him and shouting in astyle reminiscent of the Soviet era*): 'Some of you just aren't listening! That's the Soviet mentality: people don't face up to their responsibilities.'

AN ELDERLY MAN: 'It isn't easy. One can see that nothing is being done as it ought to be. It's difficult to change.'

THE *OBLAST* PUBLIC HEALTH CHIEF (*standing up at the rostrum, his tone indicating that the meeting is over*): 'He [Vladimir] is right! From now on, everyone should be taking responsibility for their behaviour. We will help those who want to get organized and they will try to convince the population . . . But I can't stand over every prostitute and make sure that she is using a condom!'

THE *OBLAST* GOVERNOR (*wrapping up in decades-old rhetorical style*): 'We understand very well that the situation is serious. Until today, we simply didn't know. But beginning now, we will take significant measure to combat this disease! Even if we can't force anyone any more . . .'

In the mid-1990s, Vladimir held the same opinions as those expressed above. But now he is firmly in the white camp, in the IDO team's eyes. To them, this change is owed to a mixture of pragmatism in the face of the conditions faced by governments in the region, and of his coming to understand the practices promoted by IDO.

Red

The second set of actors fall into the red category. As the IDO team sees it, these show the persistence of the Soviet model as the main point of reference for some local partners. The red actors are familiar with IDO's discourse and practices, but do not use this familiarity in the ways desired by the agency.

A prime example can be seen in the case of Eldar (state secretary for AIDS in a neighbouring country, like his counterpart Vladimir) and a new local NGO called Didam. Eldar exemplifies the government actors who remain stuck in their attitudes despite IDO's work, but use their familiarity with IDO's discourse to shore up their own positions on HIV/AIDS. As before, I present their debates at length in order to show the range of the different actors' thoughts, as well as their underlying agendas. Over the years, the actors have come to know the ideas of their interlocutors well, and this can be seen in their debates as they push their questioning of these ideas ever further.

One day in 1998, Anna and Beth announce to Eldar that IDO is going to disburse a large part of its budget to local NGOs. They also explain the conditions which the country will have to meet to receive aid. Eldar is furious. He insists that the non-profit nucleus forming around his arch-rival, Tatiana, is nothing but a pack of scoundrels. He scowls at the mere mention of her as if he had just been through an acrimonious divorce. The idea that other actors than himself and his subalterns could have a role in fighting the epidemic is not only inconceivable but a form of *lèse-majesté*. His attempts to incorporate the new international guidelines are desultory, and he quickly reverts to a more familiar command style.

ELDAR: 'Totally unacceptable! You should be giving me all the money, because as state secretary for AIDS, I'm the only one working in this field!'

ANNA: 'As we've already said, we are also going to finance NGOs.'

ELDAR: 'There are no NGOs working on AIDS in this country.'

BETH: 'I know of one – Boda.'

ELDAR (*repeating his old arguments, a smile on his lips*): 'That group has no one in it who is HIV-positive! And do you know why? Because they don't know who is infected! I'm the only one with that information, because now it's confidential. So the Boda people are lying to you.'

BETH: 'We've already talked about this. It's irrelevant.'

ELDAR: 'In any case, the money for NGOs should come to the one I'm going to create.'

ANNA: 'What do you mean?'

ELDAR: 'You should be funding this group! I've read IDO's guidelines and they give priority to financing NGOs that work with people living with AIDS. [*Perfectly correct: this is one of the agency's main guidelines on development and HIV prevention.*] Okay, this type of NGO doesn't exist in the country, but it's coming together as we speak! I'm encouraging infected people to do it themselves, because I understand the importance of NGOs for "people living with HIV/AIDS!" [In stark contrast to his earlier meetings with Anna, Igor and their colleagues, Eldar has now assimilated IDO's vocabulary.] I'll put you in touch with their future president, who is ill. You'll see how much infected people are in need of money. You should fund them because it's in your guidelines. And if you don't, I'll write to Geneva and New York and denounce you to your superiors!'

ANNA: 'We'll see. There is nothing that obliges us to do it.'

ELDAR (*frowning*): 'Last year and even as recently as yesterday, the Minister of Health himself expressed his satisfaction with the national AIDS programme. But it is also of concern that certain foreign forces are trying to destabilize us ...' (*A smile.*) 'Of course I'm fully in favour of a multi-sectoral approach, so long as it's under my control.'

Two days later, Beth and Anna get a call from the NGO Boda. They have been contacted by an HIV-positive man – married, with two children – who says he was ordered by Eldar to meet with IDO and tell them he was creating an NGO for people living with HIV/AIDS. If he did not comply, Eldar threatened to expose his sero-status to his neighbours and at the factory where his wife works, her wages being the sole source of the family's income. When the man refused, Eldar had carried out the threat and 'outed' him. As a result, Beth and Anna refuse to see the 'future NGO members' that Eldar wishes them to meet, on the grounds that the NGO does not yet exist.

One year later, in 1999, a new local NGO composed of HIV-positive people is officially registered with the Ministry of Health under the name of Didam. The IDO team is delighted to hear that such an NGO has been created, and Anna, Lena and Beth go to meet them.

THE NGO PRESIDENT (*with an exhausted air*): 'We are all seropositive. We've just created an NGO, so we want you to help us.'

ANNA (*stupefied to find she recognizes his face*): 'Aren't you the head of the testing lab at the National Centre for AIDS Control?' (*The lab chief admits it, furious at being found out.*) 'And you, aren't you in charge of the telephone information line at the Centre. I think I know you too: aren't you Eldar's secretary? How is it you are both a member of this NGO and on the staff of the Ministry?'

THE PRESIDENT: 'Because there are some activities that it's better to handle as a seropositive person, like talking about one's experience on television.'

LENA (*astonished*): 'You're HIV-positive?'

ANOTHER DIDAM MEMBER (*adroitly referring to IDO's guidelines*): 'We don't have to answer your question, right?'

THE PRESIDENT (*calming down*): 'All of the infected people in this country, and those close to them, are registered with our NGO. We can help and support them!'

ANNA: 'Couldn't you do it as part of your work at the Centre?'

THE PRESIDENT: 'No, we can't. No one would listen to us if we did, whereas they will if we speak as an NGO.'

THE TELEPHONE OPERATOR (*parroting IDO discourse*): 'The Centre deals with people living with HIV/AIDS as a group, whereas in the NGO we help them as individuals.'

ANNA: 'What does that mean, exactly? How do you work? How do people get in touch with you?'

THE TELEPHONE OPERATOR: 'We don't have our own office. The Centre has put a room at our disposal so that people can come to see us. They won't speak openly to the Centre's personnel, because they don't trust them, you know . . . In contrast, they know that our work respects their anonymity.'

BETH: 'How can they tell the difference if it happens in the same building and if you are working for both the Ministry and the NGO at the same time?'

ANOTHER MEMBER: 'When someone is infected, they have to come to the Centre for their test results. The medical person who deals with their case tells them the diagnosis. But from now on, that person will tell them that they can go to the NGO in the next room. They can go back to the corridor and into the other room without anyone seeing them . . .' (*More IDO discourse.*) 'That way, we will respect the dignity of the infected people and their loved ones, and help them through this terrible challenge.'

THE PRESIDENT: 'We can also do prevention work, but we haven't any funding for it. HIV is growing significantly in this country, and if you don't finance the NGO of infected people that is forming, it will be a disaster. And it will be your fault!'

As a result of this meeting, the IDO team refuses to fund Didam, which they consider Eldar's puppet. One week later, newspapers close to the government start a hostile campaign against IDO's work in the country. They charge that the agency is throwing money at 'sexual minorities and marginal people', while leaving a group of HIV-positive people to die.

For the IDO team members, Eldar's machinations are not simply the behaviour of a single official. John, Beth, Anna, Mike and their colleagues feel that Eldar is simply doing what he would have done in the Soviet era, where such practices were common. Eldar's behaviour is representative of all the actors that the team consider to be 'red'.

As we have seen, the IDO team sees the white tendency as the result of three inter-related elements: faith in the Soviet model of HIV control, pragmatic assessment of their government's material difficulties, and understanding of the logic and practices promoted by IDO. On the red side, the practices of Eldar and the members of Didam are interpreted as stemming from the same faith, assessment and understanding, but the result is a desire to return to the Soviet system. Whether considered a driver of social change (white) or resistance to social change (red), it is the post-Soviet context with its particular political and social culture that preoccupies the IDO team. As we will see, this intricately constructed cultural explanation permits the standard critique of the West's cultural hegemony (i.e., the West's imposition of culturally inappropriate approaches) to be turned on its head: rather than ask themselves whether IDO's discourse and practices are appropriate to the region, the IDO staff use post-Soviet culture as the explanation of how (or whether) these discourses and practices are received by the region's national actors.

Grey

This last section looks at the micro-strategies of resistance that IDO's partners in the region have developed over the years, and the extent to which these are used to manipulate the agency's own discourse and practices.[1] It also examines further the 'cultural' analysis adopted by the IDO actors and the political agendas hidden behind the good governance/civil society notion promoted by IDO in the field of HIV prevention.

If we accept the judgement of the IDO team, the evolution of the attitudes of formerly hostile post-Soviet actors (i.e., hostile to the discourse and practices of the agency) can be explained by the end of the USSR's 'oppression' of civil society, which can now 'blossom' in the form of NGOs. But is this an adequate explanation of the progressive adoption, or cooptation by these actors of the agency's ideas? This adoption or cooptation relates as much to Igor – who is a member of the IDO team – as to people from governments and local NGOs such as Vladimir, Tatiana, Piotr and Eldar.

From the perspective of 'incorporation of history', to use Didier Fassin's term, we can clearly understand what is behind the approach described as white by the IDO team. In contrast to what they think, this tendency is not in *contradiction* to the Soviet legacy, but is in fact – like the red approach – anchored in and derives meaning from this legacy. We will also see that, in contrast to IDO's simplifying red/white distinction, what we are really dealing with is a plethora of local strategies which, categorized as a separate tendency, I will call 'grey'. It is this which seems to be the true motor of change rather than the red/white bipolarity perceived by the IDO actors.

This historical incorporation involves two elements. The first is what Catherine Poujol describes as a 'traumatic awakening caused by the deconstruction/reconstruction of its way of life, of thought, and of action' (2000: 121), a trauma already inflicted by Russian colonization (Poujol 1992, 1993, 2001b, 2005). The second is the 'sovietism' which Olivier Roy describes as 'a form, an apparatus, and a technique of power and social organization' (1997: 18). However, what interests us is not the impact of these two historical elements on the creation of new national identities (the focus of Poujol's and Roy's studies) but on the creation of local NGOs – and more particularly, on the capacity of local actors to respond to the normative demands of a new power structure (Hann 2002a).

Thus, to understand the 'grey' tendency, some historical background is in order. The region having been first subjected to tsarist Russian colonization in the nineteenth century, its populations had already experienced the imposition of new rules dictated by state power. Subsequently, under the Soviet regime, control over collective life was significantly increased. This was not simply a matter of announcing and enforcing rules whose essential objectives (beneath the discourse of emancipation and free choice) were to maintain a particular political system in power. Rather, the aim was to forge, from the heterogeneous populations scattered across the territory of the USSR, a new and unique society: the 'socialist' society which would henceforth be the model for the rest of the world (Colas 1992).

To construct socialism, 'the Soviet authorities explicitly adopted a number of "tasks" – to use one of Lenin's favourite words – which required total mobilization even in times of peace' (Colas 1992: 286). Driving that total mobilization was not only political conviction but terror, which struck at many different types of enemy of the regime. The 'visible' enemies were foreign soldiers and political activists opposed to the USSR. The category of 'masked enemies' was more complex: 'these are the "saboteurs" and "spies" that could be anywhere, even within the party' (ibid.: 290). Also included were

> objective enemies . . . to which the term 'enemy' does not easily apply as they are not motivated by hostility and they are not aware of the damage they did. Differentiating qualifiers such as 'parasites', 'vampires' and 'wreckers' are applied to these menacing innocents. They are condemned to be purged (*cistka*) in the interests of historical necessity.
> (ibid: 290)

Such people disrupted the functioning of the Party and damaged the unity of popular will. 'Appropriate punishments' were devised for them, from psychiatric hospitals to execution. In this hierarchical society, 'enemies of the people' were severely punished for falling short of the official norms required to construct socialism (Colas 1992). But while friend and enemy are not simple categories to apply, they are all the more difficult when norms are being created in fields and activities as varied as pedagogy, organization of agricultural collectives, clinical practice and the cultivation of cotton – and indeed, governance and HIV prevention. Certainly, the objective was to implement a theoretical plan, but how could one be sure of respecting a given rule if that rule was a moving target, one being 'invented' at all levels of daily life (Colas 1992)?

That question was a serious one for Soviet citizens in view of the potential sanctions if they got it wrong. In Soviet society, the actors learned to manage such 'free space' as existed. And although all forms of collective associations were controlled by the Party and the State, there was still a process characterized as 'recomposition of solidarity groups within the framework imposed by the system' (Roy 1999: 85). Even during Stalinism, voluntary or public associations (*obshestvennie organizatsii*) represented alternative social forms to state organizations even though they officially followed party policies and were state property. These organizations made it possible for people to articulate their own interests and even contradict official Party policy (Babajanian 2005: 266). In addition, informal social networks and solidarity groups based on relations of trust and reciprocity 'were an important social space through which individuals and groups could pursue their concerns[2] in the absence of other legitimate avenues' (Babajanian 2005: 266; Shlapentokh 1989).[3]

The question is still current in the region – even if the risks are not comparable – given the ongoing creation of new rules and ways of working under pressure from the new authorities, including the international agencies. Whether certain post-Soviet actors actually convert to new ideas or not, and do or do not create new ways of doing things, whatever results is in large part the product of this historical complexity.[4]

Some actors are always a step ahead, whether they are government officials, NGO members or locally recruited IDO staff. Examples include the courageous Slava and Alexey (from the gay NGO Sisao), the wily, cultivated and witty Vladimir (state secretary for AIDS), the hard-edged and resourceful Tatiana (from the NGO Boda) and the subtle and sensitive Igor of the IDO staff. They decide to join the 'party' in power – and IDO has a certain degree of power, as we have seen – and quickly become sufficiently familiar with the new discourse and practices, using them in their own way with craft and finesse. As Vladimir said laughingly, 'I see the benefits and the costs, the opportunities and the challenges in situations. In fact, to use IDO vocabulary, and play with it a little, 'strategic planning' is a permanent activity for us![5] No one is better than we are at making plans and twisting them to our own ends! After all, we have dozens and dozens of years of training behind us!'

Then he adds, 'In any case, we don't actually have any choice, do we? We have to move forward.' They do not act out of opportunism – far too simple a label – nor in order to become members of an elite that wishes to hold the reins of power. Rather, as highly intelligent individuals, they use and in fact inhabit new spaces while still remaining within the political boundaries drawn by the new authorities.

Others, like Eldar, cling to their position, their title and the authority bestowed upon them by their office. They never work with any initiative, unless they do so with such a heavy hand that it undermines their actions (as in Eldar's creation of the NGO Didam). Beyond their personal ambitions (political and financial), it must be remembered that 'all [Soviets] were exposed to an ideology that, even when it was patently collapsing, never abandoned its claim to ethical superiority' (Hann 2002b: 11). Many believed in it to some degree and took the Soviet system for granted. Like Eldar, they are now 'regretting the shrinking of the public sector and articulating a strongly held sense that the new regimes do not respect entitlements to which they had become accustomed under socialism' (ibid.).

A final group can be thought of as 'guardians of the plan'. They move in whatever direction their superiors in the bureaucracy indicate, and find themselves arguing first in favour of a given idea, then against it, with equal force, the latest plan always having the force of law in their minds. They 'forget' – even if they were there at the various stages of its elaboration – that a plan is above all a human invention, cobbled together by bright and inventive people like Igor, Anna, Slava, Boris, Mike, John, Vladimir, Beth, Piotr or Tatiana. Without any ideas of their own, this last group waits, pen in hand, for those of other people. Then, when implementation time arrives, they cling to the plan as if it were the Bible and, as its guardians, attempt to impose it on the people they work with. They cling through thick and thin, never slacking in their adhesion until the plan is itself officially modified by colleagues and partners.

The choices made by these actors are all rooted in the Soviet era, while at the same time reflecting free choice and the special interests that have crystallized around the issue of AIDS – a far cry from adhering to one or another side of the red/white demarcation. It is not the form of collective organization (in this case, the NGO) that determines people's engagement, as the IDO team seemed to think, but – on the contrary – engagement which will work through whatever forms are available at any given moment.

In fact, it is this creativity and diversity, both anchored in history and triggering creativity, which IDO seems to have forgotten. Far from proving the universality of civil society and its 'liberation' and 'flowering' with the fall of the USSR (with its assumption that the 'seeds' for this flowering were already in place, precisely because they are universal), the attitudes of 'whitest' post-Soviet actors spring from innate enterprise and innovation, and not from the universality of a political principle.

A final twist in the tale

This last stage of our research brings up two questions. First, why is it that Beth, Anna, Igor, Mike, John and the others, despite their familiarity with the region (some were born here), were not worried by the micro-strategies of local resistance developed by some of their partners? Second, why do the IDO actors seem to have forgotten the early stages of theoretical construction of their practices, an omission that we noted in the first chapter? The two questions seem to be explained by the same phenomenon: the way these actors unwaveringly reference their actions in the over-arching notion of good governance as propagated by the agency.

If we return for a moment to the early days of this institutional ideology at IDO, we recall that this reference to good governance stems from a particular necessity: the need to create practices to fit a totally new policy created as a reference point (or theoretical underpinning) for sustainable development. We saw how this resulted in the assumption of universality for local NGOs' role in the global response to HIV/AIDS. The task of translating initially vague guidelines into practice, on the one hand, and the IDO actors' increasing understanding of the regional context on the other, made the agency's good governance ideology a necessary reference point or justification for these actors' activities.

This justificatory reference can be found in the debates presented throughout this book. A clear example can be seen in the language Beth and Anna employ during a discussion with local government officials in an isolated Central Asian province.

BETH: 'By themselves, individuals can't make all the changes necessary to reduce the factors that make them vulnerable to HIV. Of course they need to take responsibility and try to protect themselves, but they need an environment that will help them exercise that responsibility. And that is the role of civil society organizations – they're essential for creating an open, tolerant and non-discriminatory environment, and for supporting vulnerable people and helping them access prevention and care services.'

ANNA: 'In the West and in many developing countries, NGOs have sprung up in places where, for one reason or another, governments wouldn't or couldn't take measures in favour of preventing HIV or defending the rights of people affected by the virus and the people close to them.'

A MEMBER OF A STATE HEALTH INSTITUTION: 'So they are a response to Western governments' inability to represent the people?'

BETH: 'The Soviet system considered itself the sole representative of the people, and the only one with a mandate to look after the full range of the people's needs. But in reality, it only looked after the needs of its representatives. Do you want that to happen again here? Or would you rather create a strong civil society that can counterbalance the power of the state and protect you from any possible excesses by that power?'

ANNA: 'If we are going to prevent the epidemic occurring here, we need to deal with certain factors of vulnerability. And that can't be done by state services alone – they aren't representative of civil society. Local NGOs are essential … HIV prevention efforts can be stymied by hostile state

> environments, where people don't feel they can talk about their own behaviours or the risks they are taking. By that I mean the environment that is all around us, inherited from the Soviet Union. The Soviet system regarded itself as the sole voice of the people, and the only legitimate authority to take charge of meeting people's needs. But what they really took charge of were the needs of the system's representatives. Do you want that to happen again? Or would you rather have a strong civil society which can counter-balance the power of the state and protect you from the authorities' whims?'

Looking at this discourse, one is struck by the resemblance between these arguments (in favour of NGO involvement in HIV control in Central Asia and the Caucasus) and the rising 'global civil society' project in today's international relations. Since the end of the Cold War, we have indeed witnessed the emergence of a new actor, an actor whose precise shape and contours may be disputed but whose presence is not: global civil society (Chandler 2005). For many observers of international relations, 'we are in the midst of a global "associational revolution" that may prove to be as significant to the latter twentieth century as the rise of the nation-state was to the latter nineteenth' (Salomon 1994: 109). The international agenda of good governance and liberal democracy promotion is supposed to be largely responsible for this 'associational revolution' (Atlani-Duault 2005a).

This agenda is based on a 'growing consensus on the unique values of the third sector as a vital regulatory and constraining actor, which can challenge the power monopolies and inequalities enforced and promoted by both the state and the market' (Chandler 2005: 4–5; Christenson 1997; Humes and Edward 1997). This normative project is actually clearly challenging the idea of sovereignty: 'rather than the rights of states being the founding principles of international society, it should be the rights of global citizens, given voices through global civil society' (Chandler 2005: 172). According to this point of view, creating democratic structures 'beyond the nation-state' is a greater priority than simply strengthening democratic procedures within states (Grugel 2003: 273).

Under this agenda, the NGO sector has been seen as a crucial mechanism for opening up political space and challenging state regulation in the South. However, recent research has shown the limitations of this mechanism. For example, empirical case studies have challenged the notions that NGOs and community-based (or 'grassroots') organizations can truly represent the interests of the most marginal and isolated groups; rather, these studies highlight the dependency of local NGOs on their Northern partners and donors, and the influence the Northern partners have on priorities and resource allocation (Chandler 1998; Hann and Dunn 1996; Hudock 1999). Several studies suggest that the growth of community-based organizations, dependent on external funding, 'is as much as a sign of disempowerment and new forms of dependency as any positive indication of "voice" or "participation"' (Chandler 2005: 178; Chandhoke 2002; Hann and Dunn 1996; Maina 1998; Stirrat 1996). Moreover, it must be remembered that the leaders of NGOs are not elected and, unlike governments, are not subjected to democratic accountability. 'Whatever the apparently "public" part of their funding, NGOs are fundamentally – in their administration, in their formulation of policy and above all in their recruitment and social composition – private organizations' (Copans 2006: 65).

But even if observers recognize that this emerging form of governance is 'messy and unpredictable', many still believe that 'for citizens of non-democratic regimes, transnational civil society may provide the only meaningful avenue for voice and participation in decision-making' (Edwards 2001: 4). They see global civil society as a means by which individuals may be empowered to participate in global public debates, and for the voices of formerly silent victims to be heard. In this way, state interests will no longer be the only interlocutors in the discussions and decision-making about complex issues affecting the contemporary world (Kaldor 2003: 148).

The influence of the global civil society 'project' on the IDO actors seems to be paralleled or matched by that of a particular vision of communist societies. This vision springs from the critique of totalitarianism shared by many Westerners during the Cold War. According to Ferro (1999a: 27, 1999b), in addition to a list of traits that characterize a totalitarian regime – single party, terror, cult of the leader, myth of power and in the case of the Nazis, racism – these Western observers also highlighted another phenomenon: the destruction of civil society. This trait finally supplanted terror as the central element in their definition of Soviet totalitarianism (Motyl 1992a, b, and c; Werth 1992, 1993): its 'capacity to limit all independent action, in all spheres of activity' (Rupnik 1988: 272).

According to this view, it is this propensity to break something considered part of 'human nature' which reveals the most significant facet of the Soviet regime. The fundamental, defining characteristic of Soviet-style totalitarianism was its suppression of people's capacity to form political 'space' in which they could move collectively and freely. Suppressing civil society aimed to produce 'atomized' individuals, isolated by the lack of political space and kept down by terror (Atlani-Duault 2003b, 2005b).

This vision gained even wider currency in the last years of socialism (Hann and Dunn 1996), and in particular with the Polish critique of totalitarianism, beginning with the publication of a seminal article by the Polish philosopher Leszek Kolakowski in 1973. Kolakowski put forward

> the hypothesis of a historic connection between the Marxist version of a fully realized man and the fact that in real life, communism only appears in totalitarian form, and tends to replace all civil society groups or associations with coercive organs of the state.
>
> (Colas 1992: 39)

This critique of totalitarianism became manifest in Poland with the conflict between the Communist party-state and the independent trade union movement Solidarity. From that moment, the notion of civil society permitted the critics of Soviet totalitarianism to

> analyse the dead ends and dramas of this society of 'impossible citizens', and to assign a task both to the forces fighting for their freedom and to the groups aiming to reform and eventually abolish the system by liberating civil society from the party-state or even create it in countries where it had never existed.
>
> (ibid: 41)

Understanding this double influence – global civil society and Cold War anti-Sovietism – permits us to understand the last facet in the construction of IDO's institutional ideology. The logic of the agency actors can be seen in internal documents between 1994 and 2003. A typical example says, 'after the defeat of tentative reforms in the 1960s and 1970s, it became flagrantly clear that reform of the Soviet economy requires a profound democratization of the political system. Individual and private initiatives cannot express themselves unless citizens enjoy the greatest degree of liberty. This reasoning remains current but the recent context in the region adds a new dimension to conflicts between economic reform and political reforms.'

The 'new dimension' they allude to is the fall of the USSR and the political and economic transition at work in the post-Soviet countries. As an important figure in the New York headquarters confided, repeating a view circulating among interested actors, 'the dismantling of the USSR was testimony to the end of the ideological gulf which marked the twentieth century. Today there is an almost universal consensus about the importance of a system of good governance based on a pluralist democracy, a strong civil society, and an economic system that combines efficiency and growth with equity and security.'

In other words, the fall of the USSR and the end of the Cold War signalled the victory of a particular point of view, and this victory is seen as evidence of its universality. For this victory to be complete and conclusive, it seemed necessary to demonstrate it in precisely the place where the conflict began: the former Soviet Union. Its fall was not enough; its successful conversion to 'democracy' was necessary to confirm the universality of the long-awaited 'global consensus'. Unfortunately, the post-Soviet context did not seem to furnish the necessary demonstration. As the Soviet Union fell apart, the international lending institutions (among others) put pressure on governments in the region to instil market economies by privatizing resources, and to carry out economic reform in a few short years.

Certainly, the brutal imposition of a market economy worried the agencies. 'The creation of a market economy', says a typical document, 'without measures to counterbalance its effects on society represents a threat to the social fabric of post-Soviet societies: unemployment is soaring, social security systems are being dismantled, large portions of the population have fallen into poverty, and criminality grows stronger everywhere you look'.

The social consequences of introducing the market economy imperilled the hitherto unquestioned victory over the Soviet model. The agencies believed (and continue to believe) there is a risk that opposition to the Western economic model might develop within groups that originated in the Soviet system, and that these may push for a return to the Soviet era. As one unpublished paper puts it, 'the melting away of the Communist Party and all the organizations dependent on it (trade unions, youth movements, cultural associations, etc.), without any real substitutes, created a vacuum that might easily be filled by radical or extremist organizations'.

That possibility had to be countered. As one of the IDO field workers told me, 'it is crucial to create a new framework and a new equilibrium that can peacefully resolve economic, social and political conflicts that might test already fragile societies. Democratization and the participation of civil society are not just 'safety-valves'; they also permit the creation of the consensus necessary for successful and sustainable economic reforms. Support from both the central and local levels will be needed if emerging civil societies are to invest in new non-governmental structures.'

Beyond their official discourse about democratizing the region, the role of the international agencies is to support the emergence of these new structures; '[b]e they religious, ecological, cultural or economic, they are stakeholders in a phenomenon that could result in the formation of a global civil society' – itself the guarantor of victory for a certain liberal model, both political and economic. One understands why it was so important to support local NGOs in Central Asia and the Caucasus, even if they had never existed there when IDO arrived in 1994–95. Equally, one understands why the local micro-strategies of resistance we examined earlier did not worry the IDO actors. This resistance did not strike them as a threat to what they saw as the essence of their work – the creation and reinforcement of local NGOs, and therefore of civil society as a political and economic force.

Conclusion

Tuesday, September 11, 2001. It is 9 am in New York, 3 pm in Paris and 7 pm in Central Asia. The echoes of the explosions that have shaken the United States reach the borders of the former Soviet Union. In contrast to the profound anxiety on the faces of the expatriates, the local population remains impassive.

After gazing at the debris of the twin towers, the eyes of the world turn nervously towards Central Asia, on guard for the first signs of an explosion that this time will set a whole continent ablaze. Bombarded with calls and emails from family and friends who know I am in the region, it takes me a while to make my own assessment of the situation. Perhaps I am blinded by proximity, deluded by first-hand information or deceived by the apparent authority of my own eyes, but I do not see any of the things that are frightening the people who care about me in France. No signs of general uprising in Central Asia, no bellicose passions in my local friends. On the contrary, nothing changes in their air of amused, slightly disillusioned detachment about what goes on in the West – despite the general wisdom that what happens there is so important to them in today's world.

It is not that they do not understand what is occurring, much less that events in the rest of the world do not interest them. They know very well that they are involved, and that these upheavals will have repercussions for them. They have made their own quick assessments of what is at stake. Their suspicions are not assuaged by the massive arrival of American military personnel, the setting up of military bases, and the sudden interest of the Western media in their region.

Fast-forward to 2003 when, thanks partly to the local NGOs supported by the international development agencies, the Pink Revolution breaks out in Georgia. The result is the resignation of President Eduard Shevardnadze, former First Secretary of the Communist Party who had held power since he was elected president in 1992. He is replaced by Mikheil Saakashvili, a young politician with graduate degrees from universities in the United States and France. In November 2004 comes the Orange Revolution in Ukraine, which sees local NGOs – with the backing of their Georgian colleagues – organize resistance to the results of the presidential election after a representative of the political old guard 'won' it. In a second round called after the Supreme Court annuls the election, the winner is Viktor Yushchenko, a former prime minister (1999–2001) who had become the leader of the opposition coalition. February 2005 sees the outbreak of the 'Tulip Revolution' in Kyrgyzstan. In a few short weeks, the power structure is overthrown. President Askar Akayev, who has held office since independence, flees to Moscow. In May 2005, it is Uzbekistan's turn when the citizens of the city of Andijan dare to demonstrate in support of twenty-three arbitrarily jailed citizens and express their opposition to the current regime, whose power they consider illegitimate. This time, those in power respond with violence and fierce repression is unleashed on the population. The police and military shoot hundreds of people, including children and the elderly, and even more arrests are made. The repression also falls on the NGOs, who are accused of fomenting revolution. Many are simply declared illegal, while others are made to submit to increased surveillance of their activities. Other former Soviet republics take measures to prevent the revolutionary 'epidemic' and to curb the NGOs that they consider to be the source of the epidemic. New laws, such as that passed by the Russian parliament in January 2006, are drawn up to circumscribe and control NGO activities, and efforts are made to discredit them in the eyes of the citizenry through accusations of collusion with Western intelligence services.

In some cases, these 'revolutions' might appear to have been concrete expressions of democratic aspirations and clearly bring new hope to many. Nonetheless, as this study has shown, these supposedly 'spontaneous' revolutions that have periodically held the world's attention for a few days have been long in the making. They are, in fact, the product of a long historical process, which, from the fall of the USSR to the supposed 'emergence of a new civil society', has contributed much to the reconfiguration of the region's political space.

The construction of an institutional ideology

Since the fall of the USSR, the region's inhabitants have seen their hopes dwindle and their living conditions deteriorate. They have also come to know the international development agencies, to understand their logic and to appropriate their rhetoric. Whether this appropriation was done for constructive or protective purposes, it was always done in ways different from the theoretical and practical aims of the agencies' policies and programmes. At the same time, the IDO actors have also learned from and exploited their local partners' logic and *modus operandi*, sometimes working on two fronts (through their work with the partner organizations and through the recruitment of local people). This complex situation, in which the larger agendas were less important than the thoughts, acts and daily practices of individual actors, cannot be reduced to strict dichotomies of domination and subversion, or to conflicting cultures. Rather, it reflects a multitude of processes of 'co-elaboration' of discourse and practice, which have been the focus of this study.

As we have seen, since IDO first arrived in the region, the organization constructed its institutional ideology in four stages and in accordance with two main trends. The first featured the creation of a particular interpretive framework about the role of civil society in good governance, a notion which was still in flux in 1994 and of which there was no experience in the countries of the former USSR. The responses applied to development problems by civil society conformed to a certain number of logical schemas and required standardized procedures, including massive aid to local NGOs as part of promoting good governance.

During the second stage, the IDO staff had to deal with two important characteristics of public administration in the region. The first was the quasi-absence of local NGOs at the beginning of the 1990s, a legacy of Soviet-era social control, which prohibited any form of collective movement independent of the state or the Party. The second was the powerful state systems for social control themselves. Far from being daunted by this context which a priori seemed so hostile to their objectives, IDO staff's initial contacts with local partners led to the third stage during which they went in search of anything that might resemble local NGOs in the region. What they found were three types of group. The first were former Soviet associations that had been rebaptized as NGOs. The second were actually new NGOs, some of modest size and still in the process of defining their goals, some closely linked to state structures and others frankly profit-seeking. The third type was referred to as 'embryonic' NGOs – groups of friends without formal structure or official recognition such as the gay groups still largely repressed by social and legal homophobia. This, the longest stage, was the one during which IDO's programmes of assistance visibly accelerated, and during which its advocacy for local NGOs reached its peak.

It was during the fourth and final stage that a second interpretive trend began to operate among IDO staff. A new discourse emerged, which revisited the foundations of the institutional ideology and reappraised the particular conditions operating in Central Asia and the Caucasus. Far from calling into question the supposed universality of the interpretative framework which was their reference point, IDO staff integrated these conditions into the framework as additional evidence that the framework was correct. The Soviet legacy was seen – through what I call the 'white' filter – to be driving the social change promoted by IDO, as the forces oppressed by the Soviet system liberated themselves from the 'yoke of totalitarianism' thanks to the creation of civil society. In its 'red' version, the Soviet legacy was cast as the source of local resistance, which, in turn, were integrated into the evidence base that supported the framework. That is, such resistance was a surviving remnant of the Soviet system, and confirmed the need for IDO to help local NGOs 'blossom'.

Beyond integrating the discourse and practices of their partners, IDO staff did not seem to be aware of the micro-strategies of resistance that developed locally over the years. Far from confirming the simplistic white/red dichotomy, these micro-strategies of circumvention (the local partners' diversion and subversion of IDO practices) had a 'grey' foundation. This foundation was culturally and historically determined by a particularly Soviet capacity for subverting or re-casting the rules imposed by the power structure. Individual behaviour was fragmented into as many creative strategies as there were individuals. Faced with these micro-strategies of resistance, the apparent ignorance of the staff makes sense as a final 'twist in the tale'.

Why should international development agencies have invested so much energy into supporting the emergence of an active and strong civil society since their arrival in the region? The global civil society 'project' – a favourite in the world of international relations since the end of the Cold War – is certainly part of the answer. But only part, it seems to me, and one informed by a specific interpretation of post-Soviet societies. This interpretation was clearly discernable in the advisory activities of the international agencies. In their view, the destruction of civil society was a central element in Soviet totalitarianism, characterized by its ability to limit all independent action in all spheres of activity. This impulse to crush something portrayed in retrospect as part of 'human nature' in order to maintain control was seen as the most efficient and effective characteristic of the Soviet regime. Totalitarian terror in the Soviet Union succeeded in preventing any opening of independent political space and civil society, the better to keep individuals in the atomized universe of confiscated social space.

The cultural versus the political

For the first time in the history of East–West relations, international development aid has been one of the principal vectors of massive change – change which is still under way. Through a slow subversion of longstanding forms of domination, development aid turned on its head the generally accepted logic that opposes the 'political' and the 'cultural'.

For IDO staff, a 'culturalist' explanation was useful because it preempted traditional criticisms of Western cultural hegemony. First, it presupposed that civil society is not a Western social construct but something that is 'natural' to all democratic organizations and therefore independent of any given culture where it might be applied. Second, it assumed that the form taken by civil society depends greatly on cultural context.

This opposition of nature and form is key here, in that it gave a new type of legitimacy to democratization efforts. It meant there was no imposition of a Western model; rather, what happened was that a specific culture *re-emerged* in opposition to the Soviet model which had tried to crush it. In other words, the sovietization of the region could be seen as an imposed monolithic model, whereas the advent of civil society was sovietization's organic, pluralist opposite. The development agency actors based their work on a supposedly 'universal' idea which could adapt to each and every specific context, and which could work against 'democratic centralism'. As they saw it, local NGOs in the region were not imposed from without (in other words, from the West) on minority cultures, but rather facilitated the emergence of local movements that were increasingly conscious of realities denied during the Soviet era.

This explanation legitimized the international agencies' development policies in the region, which were, *prima facie*, undertaken without hegemonic intentions. But even more importantly, it freed the agencies from responsibility for failures and delays; they could blame such problems entirely on persistent anachronisms inherited from the Soviet model. This was an impressive rhetorical feat, simultaneously ignoring the reality of post-Soviet conditions and sidestepping questions about the political implications of the problems that accompanied the 'march of progress'. It permitted the agencies to portray this victory for democracy – the emergence of local NGOs as a force capable of overturning centralized power structures – as having been brought about through culture, while at the same time absolving culture of responsibility for the slightest resistance to this movement, since such resistance could be blamed entirely on the forced social uniformity of pre-democratic days. The trick for the development agencies was to ignore cultural specifics, while spreading the notion of a culture that had been obstructed and denied.

The fall of the USSR marked the victory of a point of view formulated in the United States during the Cold War. To confirm this triumph over the defunct 'Second World', it was necessary to demonstrate victory in the place where it had been most strongly resisted: the former USSR. It was not enough for the Soviet Union to have disappeared: its defeat needed to be crowned by its *conversion*, because the very absence of the USSR left open the possibility that the universality of the long-awaited 'global consensus' might be brought into question. Yet the post-Soviet reality did not seem to fit with this triumphant interpretation of history. In fact, the social consequences of introducing a market economy and party politics actually imperilled this putative victory over the Second World. There remained (and remains) the risk that state structures might veer back towards a model of government inherited from the Soviet era. The task of the international development agencies was to thwart this possibility by building up local NGOs that would act as counter-powers to the state and as guarantors of the liberal economic and political model.

And what of the epidemic?

Following the granting of independence of Central Asia and Caucasus republics and up until the mid-1990s, public health officials in the new republics accorded minimal importance to the HIV threat. In line with this approach, only governments, or, more precisely, professionals acting for the Ministries of Health and Internal Affairs, were active in fighting drug use and the HIV virus. The personnel of these ministries followed the strategy inherited from the Soviet era, that is to say, the 'control' of individuals judged dangerous to society. When the epidemic first appeared in the region in the mid-1990s, Central Asian and Caucasus leaders began to ask for help from international humanitarian and development organizations such as IDO. No new approach to the fight against HIV infection was planned. Instead, these organizations were expected to take over the financing of the programmes previously shouldered by Moscow.

Contrary to the Central Asian and Caucasus leaders' expectations, the international aid organizations refused to play the role of mere bankers. If the IDO did decide to set up in the region to fight the HIV/AIDS epidemic, it was not to finance the purchasing of equipment to restart the mass testing programme. The organization also refused to accept financial responsibility for the salaries of ministry and detoxification centre staff: these employees were paid irregularly and had been impatiently awaiting the arrival of international aid. Finally, the IDO declined to assist in the identification and isolation of injecting drug users and persons infected with the HIV virus. In a word, the IDO refused to support a Soviet-inherited strategy whereby the state exercised strict control over individuals.

Instead, the IDO actors introduced completely new practices to the region. To give but a few examples, they worked to reform HIV/AIDS detection and treatment methods; they pushed for the decriminalization of homosexuality and organized rehabilitation programmes for injecting drug users; and they helped to set up social and psychological support networks as well as structures giving legal protection to infected persons. They were also instrumental in creating and diffusing messages aimed at preventing the spread of the disease.

But, from the beginning, this aid was characterized by one particular trend: foreign donors preferred to give directly to local NGOs working against AIDS, to the detriment of government structures. If the IDO's approach exasperated some Central Asian and Caucasus officials, financial contributions made by the IDO, combined with the governments' faith in their intelligence services meant that, until the Pink Revolution broke out in Georgia, this suspicion did not lead to any real action, aside from the usual harassment by administrative departments and the police, already familiar to NGOs in the region.

The overthrow of the Georgian government, however, provoked a change in the attitudes of many regional leaders. The suspicions they previously held metamorphosed into an outright rejection of the support of local NGOs by major international and humanitarian aid agencies. On 27 December 2003, the day following Viktor Yushchenko's election as president of Ukraine, Kazakh authorities accused international humanitarian and development aid organizations of instigating the 'coloured revolutions' by helping local NGOs to rise up against the governments in place. In 2004, during one parliamentary session, the Uzbek president, Islam Karimov, accused George Soros and various international agencies of being behind the Pink Revolution in Georgia and the Orange Revolution in Ukraine, and plotting to the same end in Uzbekistan. After these agencies had been forced out of the country, many Uzbek NGOs that had accepted international aid money were declared illegal or were required to re-register with the government, a request that most often met with refusal or increased political control or interference. Consequently, their activities on the AIDS front were forcibly brought to an end.

Among the first victims of this political jousting are the region's citizens who are living with HIV and AIDS. They find themselves trapped between two conflicting visions. The first vision adheres strictly to Soviet strategy advocating tight control of individuals' actions, and its supporters are committed to re-establishing the rigid controls of the Soviet era over intimate behaviour. The second, supported by the IDO, aims at preventing the spread of HIV through decriminalizing homosexuality, rehabilitating drug users and starting up Western-style programmes aiming to convince and support rather than punish those at high risk. In this second vision, local NGOs are favoured as better positioned to deliver programmes than the state. If the first vision seemed to lose ground in the region in the second half of the 1990s, it is now triumphantly being rebuilt on the ashes of the supposed 'revolutions' that have recently shaken the former countries of the USSR.

The situation is all the more tragic because, as the last region in the world to be affected by the epidemic, Central Asia and the Caucasus are now experiencing an explosion in new cases of full-blown AIDS. If nothing is done to halt the spread of the epidemic, hundreds of thousands of new infections are likely to occur over the next decade. Tuberculosis, the most frequent opportunistic infection associated with AIDS, is widespread – a development all the more worrying because so many new cases of the disease are drug-resistant (i.e., cannot be treated with the older generation of tuberculosis medications). It is precisely now that the transition needs to be made from prevention-based programming to integrated interventions that include technically sound, properly financed care and treatment components. In addition to prevention, serious investment in clinical interventions is now necessary. As more and more people need care and treatment, state health infrastructures will be expected to provide anti-retroviral medication, treatment of AIDS opportunistic diseases and palliative care. Properly targeted, efforts to strengthen the state health infrastructure would pay off handsomely.

Yet the reality is otherwise. On the one hand, the public health capacity to deliver care and treatment has been 'hollowed out' or dismantled partly with the approval of international organizations. On the other, activities of local NGOs supported by the same organizations have been banned, physically intimidated or put under close scrutiny by state control forces. What remain are the *apparatchiks* – in the badly tailored grey suits of old times or the informal clothing of the Western newcomers – who are committed to re-establishing the rigid controls of the Soviet era over intimate behaviour. This is a sharp blow for those who, like IDO, counted on their involvement in and identification with activities apparently unrelated to politics – programmes directed at preventing the AIDS epidemic – to support political change in the region.

And yet, it should be recognized that the IDO actors and their partners helped change the discourse of public health, and managed to put a range of prevention measures in place before the epidemic had really arrived in the region – an exceptional circumstance in public health which should not be underestimated or dismissed. That the epidemic is now implanted among certain populations does not negate this achievement. Rather, it makes it even more important that such efforts be amplified or improved, and that those partners who made a difference – particularly some of the local NGOs but also some public health workers and officials – not be abandoned at a time when their work is ever more crucial.

Notes

Introduction

1 Pink in Georgia, orange in Ukraine and yellow in Kyrgyzstan (also called in this country the 'Tulip Revolution').
2 In the following chapters we will examine whence and by which processes this relatively new idea became widely used.
3 James Ferguson's study (1990) of a development agency in Lesotho is a masterful example of this kind of work. In his book, *The Anti-Politics Machine*, Ferguson shows how the World Bank's agricultural development projects, beyond their apparent inability to meet their official goals, in reality serve to de-politicize interventions by the state without threatening its (the state's) durability. Despite their apparent inefficiency, these projects manage to establish government authority much more strongly than if their initial aims – a priori purely technical and agricultural – had achieved the original objectives. As Ferguson puts it,

> From this perspective the development machine in Lesotho is not a poverty eliminating machine which would incidentally strengthen state bureaucracy, but a machine to strengthen and spread the exercise of bureaucratic state power which happens to take 'poverty' as the starting point.
>
> (1990: 255)

4 For an analysis of 'developmental populism', see Olivier de Sardan (1995).
5 This perspective has been possible partly due to the work of Michel Foucault on the dynamics of ideas and power, and on the creation of mechanisms through which certain representations of the world have become dominant (Escobar 1996).
6 See Agier and Bouchet Soulnier 2004; Baré 1995; Bornstein 2003; Copans 2006; Crewe and Harrison 1998; Fassin 2007; Fassin and Rechtman 2007; Fassin and Vasquez 2005; Ferguson 1990; Hobart 1993; Gardner and Lewis 1996; Grillo and Stirrat 1997; Gupta 1998; Long and Long 1992; Malkki 1995; Marie 2005; Mosse 2005; Olivier de Sardan 1995; Pandolfi 2003; Pottier 1997, Quarles Van Ufford and Giri 2003; Redfield 2005; Seidel and Vidal 1997; Shore and Wright 1997; Vidal 2004. These references are not, of course, exhaustive.
7 Olivier de Sardan refers to 'developmentalist configuration' as a 'complex group of institutions, of influx and of actors, for whom development constitutes a resource, a career, a market, a stake or a strategy' (2002: 731).
8 This approach was not the only one I could have chosen. For an overview of the richness and diversity of ethnographic methods used to study development and HIV/AIDS, see Parker and Ehrhardt 2001.
9 Internal literature, unpublished and not referenced.

1 The first steps

1 Bruno Lautier, for example, examines the use of the term governance in the World Bank's new stance on the fight against poverty and notes that for the World Bank, economics became little by little a 'moral science' during the 1990s (2001: 69).
2 For example, an IDO project for the promotion of good governance in the East, a World Bank project on the fight against malaria in India, a programme of structural adjustment put into place by the IMF in Argentina and so on.
3 Depending on the projects, the putative beneficiaries are the populations affected by development activities (for example: the Indians in the project area of the World Bank's programme to fight malaria, the Argentineans in the IMF's structural adjustment programme, etc.).
4 International actors include multilateral agencies such as IDO, the Organization for Security and Co-operation in Europe (studied by Berg and Kreikemeyer 2006b) and bilateral agencies (USAID, DFID, GTZ, etc., see de Martino 2005 for a study of Swiss assistance to Central Asia), and a range of international NGOs. These run the gamut from Médecins du Monde and Soros Foundation/Open Society Institute (OSI) to Turkish NGOs (particularly active upon the educational system, see Demir, Balci and Akkok 2000) and Christian NGOs, whose humanitarian activities go hand in hand with their missionary work.
5 In fact, the true beneficiaries of the 'green revolution' were above all big landowners, who were the only ones with the means to make the necessary investments in technology.
6 Cf. for example, Raul Prebisch (1950).
7 For more details, see for example, International Labour Organization (1976).
8 See for example, UNICEF (1991).
9 *Managing development: the governance dimension*, working document eventually published as *Governance and development*, Washington D.C.: World Bank, 1992.
10 Most of this is 'grey literature' or non-published documents. The unreferenced quotations in this chapter come from such documents.
11 For a review of the literature on the extraordinary movement of NGOs in the fight against HIV in the world, see for example, Aggleton 1989; Aggleton and Homans 1988; Aggleton *et al.* 1992, 1993; Altman 1994; Barnett and Blaikie 1992; Bolton 1992; Bolton *et al.* 1991; Kalibala *et al.* 1997; Kramer 1988; Mann *et al.* 1995; Parker 1996.
12 The term 'patient empowerment' came out of the struggle in the United States for recognition of the rights and capabilities of sick people to take control of their destiny.
13 One of the first NGOs active in the fight against the epidemic in Uganda, TASO was founded in 1987 by Noerine Kaleeba, the widow of the first Ugandan to openly acknowledge having AIDS. TASO brought together HIV-positive people and members of their families and friends in an organization which became a model for many others in Africa and elsewhere (Kalibala, Rubaramira and Kaleeba, 1997: 5155).
14 In a large number of cities worldwide, the development of gay organizations over the past years was greatly encouraged by the HIV/AIDS epidemic. It aroused a sense of urgency while gathering the resources necessary for an organized fight (Miller 1992). Groups such as Pink Triangle in Kuala Lumpur, the Bombay Dost in India, Proyecto Germinal in Lima or the Library Foundation in the Philippines created a concrete link between the prevention of HIV among gays and the public emergence of a homosexual community; the space opened by the fight against HIV served the two objectives at the same time. HIV/AIDS also prompted the

creation of associations of prostitutes. An example is Patita Uddhar Sabha, founded in 1992 by the prostitutes of an area in New Delhi, which carries out prevention activities and advocates better health services from the Indian government (Dhawan and Narula 1992).

15 This step of home help was adopted due to and during the same period by numerous associations surrounding the elderly, and on the same 'anti-institutional' theme.

16 See also Adam *et al.* 1999; Dowsett 1996; Parker 1990, 1996.

2 The legacy

1 For a bibliography, see, among others, Abramson 1999; Allworth 1989; Atabaki and O'Kane 1999; Babajanian 2005; Babajanian, Freizer and Stevens 2005; Banuazizi 1994; Belenitsky 1968; Berg 2002, 2003; Berg and Kreikemeyer 2006; Berton-Hogge 1992; Braud 1993; Brill Olcott 1987; Broers 2005; Brown 1998; Cagnat and Jan 1990; Carrère d'Encausse 1978, 1990, 1991, 1992; Charachidzé 1989; Chuvin 2004; Chuvin and Gentelle 1998; Critchlow 1991; Dawisha and Parrott 1994, 1997; Djalili and Kellner 2001; Earle 2004, 2005; Elleinstein 1992; Everett-Heath 2003; Ferro 1993, 1999a and b; Fourniau 1994; Freizer 2005; Howell 1996; Hyman 1994; Ilkhamov 2005; Kandiyoti 1996, 2002, 2004; Kandiyoti and Mandel 1998; Kuehnast 1998; Kulchik, Fadin and Sergeyev 1996; Laruelle 2004; Levitin 2001; Luong-Jones 2002, 2004; Luong-Jones and Weinthal 1999; Mandel 2002; Mandelbaum 1994; Mandrillon 1992; Massicard and Trevisani 2003; Melvin 2000; Motyl 1992a, b and c; Olcott 2002; Paksoy 1994; Petric 2002, 2005; Peyrouse 2004; Poujol 1992, 1993, 1997, 2000, 2001a and b, 2005; Raballand 2005; Radvanyi 1990, 1993, 1997, 2003; Rashid 1994; Rasizade 2002; Romer *et al.* 1992; Roux 1997; Roy 1992a and b, 1997, 1999, 2001, 2002; Ruffin and Waugh 1999; Rumer 1989, 1996; Sapir 1993a, b and c; Schoeberlein 1999, 2000a, 2000b, 2002; Sievers 2003; Stevens 2005; Urjewwick 1993; Werner 1998.

2 National Statistics Committee of the Kyrgyz Republic (2000).

3 In the domain of education, every child in school completed free compulsory education and the state paid for textbooks, school uniforms and free hot meals up till the fourth grade. At the time of independence, Central Asia's adult literacy level of 98.4 per cent was similar to that of advanced industrial countries (UNDP 1999a).

4 In the Kyrgyz republic, for example, industrial output fell by 70 per cent during the first five years after independence (UNDP 1999a: 9). Between 1991 and 1999, in the most heavily industrialized country of the region, Kazakhstan, the share of industry in GDP fell from 30 per cent to 20 per cent (UNDP 1999a).

5 Although Rasizade is describing Azerbaijan, the same situation was shared by all.

6 For detailed studies on how people have coped with the decline of public services and, more generally, with the dramatic changes in post-Soviet economies, see the special issue of *Central Asian Survey* devoted to market reforms, social dislocations and survival in post-Soviet Central Asia, edited by Deniz Kandiyoti and Ruth Mandel (1998). See for example Kandiyoti's excellent analysis showing how rural households in the Andijian province of eastern Uzbekistan responded to the transformations in their livelihoods (1998), Werner's study of a collective farm in South Kazakhstan Oblast (1998), Harris' study of how people cope with daily life in some Tajik villages (1998), and Brown (1998), Howell (1996) and Kuehnast's (1998) articles on the diversity of coping strategies in Kazakhstan and Kyrgyzstan.

7 The environmental situation does not help. During the Soviet period, hundreds of nuclear, chemical and biological weapon tests were conducted in Central Asia,

mainly in Semipalatinsk (Kazakhstan), Naryn (Kyrgyzstan) and on Resurrection Island (Kazakhstan and Uzbekistan). There is evidence that in the course of some of these tests, radiation and chemicals made their way to human settlements close to the test ranges (Sievers 2003: 33). Facilities for the actual production of chemical and biological weapons, including for the production of anthrax, were located in Karakalpastan (Uzbekistan) and Stepnogorsk (Kazakhstan).

8 BSS (behavioural surveillance) provides evidence of this and many studies have been done in Central Asia since 2000, but relatively few are published.

9 Cited by *Russia Today Online* (28 April 1999).

10 In Kyrgyzstan, behavioural surveys carried out in 2000 found that:

> 96 per cent of drug users share syringes, 99 per cent inject drugs with a syringe from a common container, 35 per cent use one syringe more than 20 times; 42 per cent share syringes; 64 per cent cannot afford to buy syringes; and only 14 per cent use sterile syringes.
>
> (Godinho *et al.* 2004: 51)

11 For a review of literature on sexuality, contraception and policies in the field of family planning and public health in the time of the USSR and during the post-Soviet years, see for example, Adeyi *et al.* 1997; Afanasyev and Skorobogatov 1996; Avdeev *et al.* 1994; Blum 1994; Bobak *et al.* 1998; Boekham and Zmushko 1998; Chaika *et al.* 1991; Davies 1989, 1990, 1993; Kon 1989, 1991, 1992, 1995; Kon and Riordan 1993; Linglof 1995; Riordan 1990; Williams 1995. However, these studies focus on Russia and the European part of the old Soviet Empire and not on the countries of Central Asia and the Caucasus.

12 For a study of Uzbekistan, see Buckley, Barrett and Asminkin 2004.

13 On this question, see Barnett *et al.* 2004.

14 The reference study on bridging populations is that of Morris *et al.* (1996). It shows that men who had sexual relations with both their usual partners and prostitutes have contributed significantly to the explosion of the epidemic in Thailand.

15 See Davies 1983, 1984, 1987, 1988, 1989, 1990, 1993; Field 1957, 1976; Hyde 1974; Kaser 1976; Knaus 1982; Lisitsyn 1972; Navarro 1977; Ryan 1978, 1987, 1991; Safonov and Loginova 1976; Serenko *et al.* 1976.

16 The strategy of mass testing chosen in the USSR differed greatly from that of the United Nations. The following is from the official position of WHO:

> Mandatory testing does not promote safer behaviour and impedes behavioural counselling. The evidence that voluntary HIV testing leads to safer behaviour is weak, but even if this was clearly demonstrated; it would be illogical to conclude that compulsory testing would have the same effect. It is paradoxical to try to gain people's voluntary co-operation on adopting safer behaviour by coercing them to be tested ... Mandatory testing erodes the basis of trust between health service providers or government authorities and people who would otherwise benefit from health services. It can damage the public health by deterring people from using health services from which they or their families would otherwise benefit.
>
> (WHO 1993: 8–9)

17 The position of WHO on contact tracing and HIV is the following:

> The aim of contact tracing for curable sexually transmitted diseases is to identify and treat possibly infected contacts, to prevent them from developing future disease and to break the chain of transmission. This is not possible for HIV because there is no cure. Contact tracing or partner notification

> of HIV is, on balance, desirable to enable contacts to be aware of the extent to which they have been at risk, and to offer voluntary testing and care if found to be infected. But the public health benefits of contact tracing for HIV are much more doubtful and equivocal than that for, say, syphilis or gonorrhoea.
>
> (WHO 1993: 40)

18 Just before the collapse of the USSR, the territory contained 1,500 HIV diagnostic laboratories and 110 'prevention' centres (15 at the Republic level, 6 at the Russian Federation regional level, and 89 in the Soviet Republics, *oblasts* and principal towns). In 1988, 600 doctors were trained in HIV laboratory diagnostics and 890 in clinical treatment. One year later there were 1,420 and 1,600 respectively (Williams 1995).

3 Negotiating assistance

1 Saltmarshe (1996: 395) notes that, at the beginning of international organizations' interventions, 'non-governmental activity is frequently misunderstood as being anti-governmental activity'.
2 See for example, Moatti and Souterrand (2000).
3 Beth is referring to a notion that is in vogue in scientific and NGO circles at the time, that of 'vulnerability' to HIV.
4 This is a reference to current agency discourse about the relationship between development and the 'capacity to choose'.
5 For the study of a discourse linking the issues of human rights and democratization in Central Asia see Berg and Kreikemeyer (2006a and 2006b) and their study of the OSCE 'ODHIR Human Rights Monitoring and Reporting Training'.
6 The Government Organized NGO (GONGO) phenomenon in the region has been studied by, among others, Babajanian 2005; Berg 2003; Ilkhamov 2005; Mandel 2002; and Sievers 2003.
7 For studies of the DONGO phenomenon in Central Asia, see, for example, Berg 2003; Ilkhamov 2005; Kandiyoti 2004; Mandel 2002; Sievers 2003; Stevens 2005.
8 In certain countries, gay NGOs were and are still among the most active groups in developing HIV/AIDS prevention activities. As mentioned previously, the first group of gay HIV activists was GMHC (Gay Men's Health Crisis), founded in New York in 1982. Faced with the need to put in place quickly a multitude of direct support services for HIV-positive people, the movement set up voluntary programmes for home care and support. These activities were quickly taken up by groups in other American cities, and then by similar movements in other parts of the world. There are numerous examples in New Zealand, where the first support network was set up by a small group of gay men; in Britain, where friends founded the Terrence Higgins Trust after Higgins died (Davies *et al.* 1993); in Sweden and Denmark, where existing gay associations took on the challenge of HIV/AIDS despite tensions between two of them (Altman 1994). In Latin America as well, the influence of gay men was significant. In countries such as Peru, Mexico and Nicaragua, gay movements played key roles in the creation of specific AIDS-related organizations (with, at least in Peru and Nicaragua, the participation of lesbian groups). In Chile, the first anti-AIDS NGO was the *Corporación Chileña de Prevención del SIDA*, founded by a group of gay friends. In Brazil, gay groups got involved with social workers, researchers, progressive clergy and HIV-positive people to start such organizations (Altman 1994; Parker 1990). Gay groups in Malaysia (e.g., Pink Triangle) and Singapore played key roles in the creation of the first anti-AIDS organizations, and were influential in India, Hong Kong, Japan, Indonesia and the Philippines.

9 Useful information on this subject can be found in Robinson (1993).
10 Although not involved in the trainings described here, INTRAC publications (such as Buxton 2004; Garbutt and Heap 2003; Giffen, Earle and Buxton 2005; Heap *et al.* 2000; Hunt 2001) provide insight into how a major UK NGO that has been providing management and policy trainings to Central Asian NGO leaders since the mid-1990s sees its local partners in the region. Also from INTRAC, for very interesting analysis of the complex and varied nature of possible partnerships between Northern and Southern NGOs, see James (2001); Brehm, Harris-Curtis *et al.* (2004); Mawdsley, Townsend, Porter and Oakley (2002). Finally, from this same team and more specifically about the AIDS issue (but not about the region described in this book), James (2005) looks at the way approaches to organizational capacity building could help NGOs to effectively respond to the epidemic.
11 There were about 25,000 in the entire country at the time.
12 In Central Asia, Soros/OSI has also done superb work among injecting drug users: see Malinowska-Sempruch (2002); Malinowska-Sempruch and Gallagher (2004) for further information.

4 White, red and grey

1 Micro-resistance refers to hidden forms of resistance in everyday life – the 'weapons of the weak' as Scott put it (1985, 1990). Scott showed how, in the guise of submission, subordinate groups develop 'hidden transcripts' that criticize authority without the latter being aware of it (1990: xii).
2 With, for example, 'protest letters, dissemination of suppressed literature (*samizdat*), organized actions and political gatherings, *bard* movements, informal or dissident movements and support for political activist and dissidents' (Babajanian 2005: 266).
3 This so-called Soviet 'economy of favours' was described in detail by Ledeneva (1998).
4 There is a growing literature documenting various communal forms of social organization and processes of civic life in post-Soviet Central Asia and the Caucasus. See among others Akiner (2002); Babajanian (2005); Babajanian, Freizer and Stevens (2005); Berg (2003); Broers (2005); Earle (2005); Freizer (2005); Kandiyoti (1998); Ilkhamov (2005); Petric (2002, 2005); Poujol (2001a); Stevens (2005); Roy (1999).
5 Vladimir is playing with a term that has become very current, almost 'politically correct', at IDO and the other international agencies in recent years. All planning now has to be 'strategic' and all local partners like Vladimir working in HIV prevention have been obliged to take training sessions on strategic planning.

Bibliography

Abramson, D. (1999) 'A critical look at NGOs and civil society as means to an end in Uzbekistan', *Human Organization*, 58(30): 240–50.

Adam, B. A., Duyvendak, J. W. and Krouvel, A. (1999) *The Global Emergence of Gay and Lesbian Politics. National Imprints of a Worldwide Movement*, Philadelphia, PA: Temple University Press.

Adeyi, O. (2003) *Averting AIDS crises in Eastern Europe and Central Asia: a regional support strategy*, Washington DC: World Bank.

Adeyi, O., Chellaraj, G., Goldstein, E., Preker, A. and Ringold, D. (1997), 'Health Status during the Transition in Central and Eastern Europe: Development in Reverse', *Health Policy and Planning*, 12(2): 132–45.

Afanasyev, V. and Skorobogatov, S. (1996) 'Prostitution in St. Petersburg', in M. Jyrkinen (ed.) *Conference Book: Changing Faces of Prostitution Conference, Helsinki, 3–5 May 1995*, Helsinki: Unioni, The League of Finnish Feminists.

Aggleton, P. (1989) 'Evaluating Health Education about AIDS', in P. Aggleton, G. Hart and P. Davies (eds) *AIDS: Social Representations, Social Practices*, London: Falmer Press.

Aggleton, P. and Homans, H. (eds) (1988) *Social Aspects of AIDS*, London: Falmer Press.

Aggleton, P., Hart, G. and Davies, P. (1992) *AIDS: Rights, Risk and Reason*, London: Falmer Press.

—— (1997) *AIDS: Activism and Alliances*, London: Taylor and Francis.

—— (1999) *Families and Communities. Responding to AIDS*, London: Taylor and Francis.

Aggleton, P., Weeks, J. and Taylor-Laybourn, A. (1993) 'Voluntary Sector Responses to HIV and AIDS: a Framework for Analysis', in P. Aggleton, G. Hart and P. Davies (eds) *AIDS: Facing the Second Decade*, London: Falmer Press.

Agier, M. and Bouchet Saulnier, F. (2004) 'Humanitarian Spaces: Spaces of Exception' in F. Weisman (ed.) *In the Shadow of 'Just Wars'*, New York: Cornell University Press.

Akiner, S. (2002) 'Prospects for civil society in Tajikistan', in A. Sajoo (ed.) *Civil Society in the Muslim World: Contemporary Perspectives*, London: I.B. Tauris.

Allworth, E. (ed.) (1989) *Central Asia: a Century of Russian Rule*, Durham, NC: Duke University Press.

Altman, D. (1994) *Power and Community: Organizational and Cultural Responses to AIDS*, London: Taylor and Francis.

Anonymous (2003) 'Health and dictatorship: effects of repression in Turkmenistan', *The Lancet*, 361: 69–70.

Apthorpe, R. (1997) 'Writing development policy and development analysis plain or clear: on language, genre and power', in S. Shore and S. Wright (eds) *Anthropology of policy: critical perspectives on governance and power*, London: Routledge.

Apthorpe, R. and Gasper, D. (eds) (1996) *Arguing development policy: frames and discourses*, London: Frank Cass.

Aral, S. O. and St. Lawrence, J. S. (2002) 'The Ecology of Sex Work and Drug Use in Saratov, Russia', *Sexually Transmitted Diseases*, 29(12): 798–805.

Aral, S. O., St. Lawrence, J. S., Tikhonova, L., Safarova, E., Parker, K. A., Shakarishvili, A. and Ryan, C. A. (2003) 'The Social Organization of Commercial Sex Work in Moscow, Russia', *Sexually Transmitted Diseases*, 30(1): 39–45.

Arce, A. (2003) 'Value contestations in development interventions: community development and sustainable livelihoods approaches', *Community Development Journal*, 38(3): 199–212.

Arce, A. and Long, A. (2000) *Anthropology, development and modernities: exploring discourses, counter-tendencies and violence*, London: Routledge.

Armenian National AIDS Centre (2005) 'HIV/AIDS epidemic in the Republic of Armenia', Fact sheet, Yerevan.

Atabaki, T. and O'Kane, J. (1999) *Post-Soviet Central Asia*, London: Tauris.

Atlani, L. [see also Atlani-Duault] (1997) 'Assistance aux victimes de violences sexuelles dans les camps de réfugiés. Ethnographie d'une politique', *Psychopathologie africaine*, XXVIII(1): 25–53.

—— (1998) 'Le sida se lève à l'Est', *Transcriptase. Revue critique de l'actualité scientifique internationale sur le VIH et les virus des hépatites*, 64: 20–24.

—— (2002) 'Europe de l'Est: aujourd'hui, les usagers de drogues. Et demain?', *Trancriptase. Revue critique de l'actualité scientifique internationale sur le VIH et lesvirus des hépatites*, 100: 67–68.

Atlani, L. and Rousseau, C. (2000) 'The Politics of Culture in Humanitarian Aid to Refugees Having Experienced Sexual Violence', *Transcultural Psychiatry*, 37(3): 435–49.

Atlani, L., Caraël, M., Brunet, J. B., Frasca, T. and Chaika, N. (2000) 'Social Change and AIDS in the Former Soviet Union: the Making of an Epidemic', *Social Sciences and Medicine*, 50: 1547–56.

Atlani-Duault, L. [see also Atlani] (2003a) 'Les ONG locales, vecteurs de 'bonne gouvernance' dans le Second Monde? Introduction à une étude de cas', *Le Journal des anthropologues*, 94–95: 183–90.

—— (2003b) 'La 'bonne gouvernance', nouvelle éthique du développement? Quelques propositions pour une réflexion critique', *Autrepart*, 28: 165–80.

—— (2005a) (ed.) *Les ONG à l'heure de la 'bonne gouvernance'*, Paris: Armand Colin / Autrepart, Special issue, 35: 184.

—— (2005b) *Au bonheur des autres. Anthropologie de l'aide humanitaire*, Nanterre: Société d'ethnologie.

—— (2006a) 'Comment se créent les normes. De la prévention des conflits aux révolutions en ex-URSS', in N. Bagayoko-Penone and B. Hours (eds) *États, ONG et Production des normes sécuritaires dans les pays du Sud*, Paris: L'Harmattan.

—— (2006b) 'Entre mémoire et oubli: la construction institutionnelle de la souffrance sociale. Essai d'anthropologie politique de l'aide au développement', in J. F. Baré (ed.) *Paroles d'expert*, Paris: Karthala.

—— (2007) "Revolutions' clothed in the colors of spring. Exporting democracy to the East', in M. Feher (ed.) *Non-Governmental Politics*, New York: Zone Books.
—— (forthcoming) 'Sur les cendres des révolutions de couleur. Drogues et Démocratisation en Asie Centrale post-soviétique', *Revue d'études comparatives Est-Ouest*.
Augé, M. (1983) 'Ordre biologique, ordre social. La maladie comme forme élémentaire de l'événement', in M. Augé and C. Herzlich (eds) *Le sens du mal. Anthropologie. Histoire, sociologie de la maladie*, Paris: Éditions des Archives contemporaines.
—— (1986) 'L'anthropologie de la maladie', in *Anthropologie. État des lieux*, Paris: Éditions de l'EHESS / Librairie générale française.
Avdeev, A., Blum, A. and Trotiskaya, I. (1994) 'Histoire de la statistique de l'avortement en Russie et en URSS', *Population*, 4–5: 903–35.
Babajanian, B. (2005) 'Civic participation in Post-Soviet Armenia', *Central Asian Survey*, 24(3): 261–79.
Babajanian, B., Freizer, S. and Stevens, D. (2005) 'Introduction: Civil society in Central Asia and the Caucasus', *Central Asian Survey*, 24(3): 209–24.
Banégas, R. and Meyer, P. (2002) 'La gouvernance, un concept 'attrape-tout' transversal et fluctuant': unpublished.
Banuazizi W. (1994) *The New Geopolitics of Central Asia and its Borderlands*, London: Tauris.
Baré, J.-F. (ed.) (1995) *Les applications de l'anthropologie. Un essai de réflexion collective depuis la France*, Paris: Karthala.
—— (2001) 'L'évaluation de l'intervention publique comme exercice d'anthropologie historique', in J.-F. Baré (ed.) *L'évaluation des politiques de développement. Approches pluridisciplinaires*, Paris: L'Harmattan.
Barnett, T. and Blaikie, P. (1992) *AIDS in Africa: Its Present and Future Impact*, London: Belhaven Press.
Barnett, T. and Whiteside, A. (1997) 'The Social and Economic Impact of HIV/AIDS in Ukraine', British Council report, Ukraine: unpublished.
—— (2002) *AIDS in the Twenty-first Century: Disease and Globalisation*, London: Palgrave.
Barnett, T., Ivanov, A. and Slay, B. (eds) (2004) *HIV and Human Development in Central and Eastern Europe and the Commonwealth of Independent States, Reversing the Epidemic, Facts and Policy Options*, New York: UNDP.
Barnett, T., Whiteside, A., Khodakevich, L., Kruglov, Y. and Steshenko, V. L. (2000) 'The HIV/AIDS Epidemic in Ukraine: its Potential Social and Economic Impact', *Social Science and Medicine*, 51(9): 1387–403.
Barowitz, M., Lowndes, C. M., Garnett, G., Grassly, N., Rhodes, T. and Stimson, G. V. (2001) 'Intersecting Epidemics and Linked Responses: HIV and STI in the Former Soviet Union', *International Journal of STD and AIDS*, 12 (sup. 2): 10.
Belenitsky, A., (1968) *Asie centrale*, Genève: Nagel.
Bellier, I. and Wilson, T. (eds) (2000) *An Anthropology of the European Union: Building, Imagining, Experiencing Europe*, Oxford: Berg.
Berg, A. (2002) 'Local vs. Global Concepts of Gender Complicate NGO Work in Uzbekistan', *Give & Take*, 2–3: 22–23.
—— 2003, 'Encountering Transition in Contemporary Uzbekistan – A Critical Perspective on Foreign Aid and Non-Governmental Organizations', in M. Dreger and A. Huenninghaus (eds) *Social Research on Transformation in Developing*

Countries–Results of Interdisciplinary PhD-school Participants, Bochum 2003 (IEE Working Paper 171).
Berg, A. and Kreikemeyer, A. (eds) (2006) *Realities of Transformation. Democratization Policies in Central Asia Revisited*, Baden-Baden: Nomos.
Berton-Hogge, R. (ed.) (1992) *La fin de l'URSS. Héritages d'un empire*, Paris: La Documentation française.
Bibeau, G. (1996) 'La spécificité de la recherche anthropologique sur le sida', in J. Benoist and Alice Desclaux (eds), *Anthropologie et sida: Bilan et perspectives*, Paris: Karthala, 13–30.
Bisiou, Y. (2004) 'Drogue: une prohibition sous influence', *Transcriptase. Revue critique de l'actualité scientifique internationale sur le VIH et les virus des hépatites*, 116: 33–35.
Blomstrom, M. and Hettne, B. (1984) *Development Theory in Transition*, London: Zed Books.
Blum, A. (1994) *Naître, vivre et mourir en URSS*, Paris: Plon.
Blundo, G. (2000) 'Élus locaux et courtiers en développement au Sénégal: trajectoires politiques, modes de légitimation et stratégies d'alliance' in J.P. Olivier de Sardan, T. Biershenk and J.P. Chauveau (eds) *Courtiers en développement. Les villages africains en quête de projets*, Paris: Karthala.
Bobak, M., Pickhart, H., Hertzman, C., Rose, R. and Marmot, M. (1998) 'Socio-Economic Factors, Perceived Control and Self-Reported Health in Russia. A Cross-Sectional Survey', *Social Sciences and Medicine*, 47(2): 269–79.
Boekham, V. and Zmushko, E. I. (1998) 'Home-made Drugs as an Active Factor for HIV Transmission in Russia', paper presented at the 12th World AIDS Conference, Geneva, July.
Bolton, R. (1992) 'Mapping Terra Incognita: Sex Research for AIDS Prevention. An Urgent Agenda for the 1990s', in G. Herdt and S. Lindenbaum (eds) *The Time of AIDS. Social Analysis, Theory and Method*, Newbury Park, CA: Sage Publications.
Bolton, R., Lewis, M. and Ayoma, O. B. (1991) 'AIDS Literature for Anthropologists: a Working Bibliography', *Journal of Sex Research*, 28(2): 307–46.
Borisenko, K., Tichonova, L. I. and Renton, A. M. (1999) 'Syphilis and Other Sexually Transmitted Infections in the Russian Federation', *International Journal of STD and AIDS*, 10: 665–68.
Bornstein, E. (2003) *The Spirit of Development: Protestant NGOs, Morality and Economics in Zimbabwe*, London: Routledge.
Bourgeois, P. (1995) *In Search of Respect: Selling Crack in El Barrio*, Cambridge: Cambridge University Press.
Braud, D. (1993) *L'expérience soviétique et sa remise en cause*, Paris: Dalloz / Sirey.
Brehm, V., Harris-Curtis, E., Padrão, L. and Tanner, M. (2004) *Autonomy or Dependence: Case Studies of North-South NGO Partnerships*, Oxford: INTRAC Publications.
Brill Olcott, M. (1987) *The Kazakhs*, Stanford, CT: Hoover Institution.
—— (1996) *Central Asia's New States. Independence, Foreign Policy and Regional Security*, Washington DC: United States Institute of Peace Press.
Brill Olcott, M. and Udalova, N. (2000) 'Drug Trafficking on the Great Silk Road: the Security Environment in Central Asia', Working Paper No. 11, Washington DC, Carnegie Endowment for International Peace: unpublished.
Broers, L. (2005) 'After the "revolution": civil society and the challenge of consolidating democracy in Georgia', *Central Asian Survey*, 24(3): 333–50.

Brown, A. J. (1998) 'Taking shelter: the art of keeping a roof overhead in post-Soviet Almaty', *Central Asian Survey*, 17(4): 613–28.

Brown, P. J. (1998) *Understanding and Applying Medical Anthropology*, London: Mayfield.

Brunet, J. B. (1997) 'Monograph on HIV Infection in Russia', UNAIDS report: unpublished.

Buckley, C. J. (1997) 'Suicide in Post-Soviet Kazakhstan: Role Stress, Age and Gender', *Central Asian Survey*, 16(1): 45–52.

—— (2002) 'Children at Risk: Child Health in Central Asia', William Davidson Institute Working Papers, No. 523.

—— (2005a) 'Migration, Family Networks, and HIV Risk: Insights from the Caucasus' *Conference proceedings. Women Migrants and HIV/AIDS in the World: An Anthropological Approach*, Paris: UNESCO.

—— (2005b) 'The Socio-Cultural Correlates of HIV/AIDS in the Southern Caucasus' in *The Social and Cultural Context of HIV/AIDS in the Caucasus*, Paris: UNESCO.

Buckley, C. J., Barrett, J. B. and Asminkin, Y. P. (2004) 'Reproductive and Sexual Health Among Young Adults in Uzbekistan', *Studies in Family Planning*, 35(1): 1–14.

Burawoy, M., Blum, J. A., George, S., Gille, Z., Gowan, T., Haney, L., Klawiter, M., Lopez, S. H., Riain, S. O. and Thayer, M. (2000) *Global Ethnography: Forces, Connections, and Imaginations in a Postmodern World*, Berkeley, CA: University of California Press.

Burgasov, N. P. (1986) 'Vistuplenye na kruglom stole', *Literaturnaya gazeta*, 7: 15.

Buxton C. (2004) *Who Benefits? The Monitoring and Evaluation of Development Programmes in Central Asia*, Oxford: INTRAC Publications.

Cagnat, R. and Jan, M. (1990) *Le milieu des empires, entre URSS, Chine et Islam: le destin de l'Asie centrale*, Paris: Robert Lafont.

Carothers, T. (1999) *Aiding democracy abroad. The learning curve*, Washington DC: Carnegie Endowment for International Peace.

Carrère d'Encausse, H. (1978) *L'empire éclaté: la révolte des nations en URSS*, Paris: Le Seuil.

—— (1981) *Réforme et Révolution chez les musulmans de l'Empire Russe,* 2nd edition, Paris: Presses de la Fondation Nationale des Sciences Politiques.

—— (1990) *L'empire éclaté: la révolte des nations en URSS*, Paris: Librairie générale française.

—— (1991) *La gloire des nations ou La fin de l'empire soviétique*, Paris: Fayard.

—— (1992) 'Cela s'appelait l'URSS, et après . . . ', *Hérodote*, 64: 3–219.

Cattachin, S., Panchaud, C. and Tattini, V. (1996) *Les politiques de lutte contre le VIH/SIDA en Europe de l'Ouest. Du risque à la normalisation*, Paris: L'Harmattan.

Center for Disease Control / Central Asia Region (CDC/CAR) (2002) 'HIV and AIDS Epidemic in Central Asia', report: unpublished.

Chaika, N. A. *et al.* (1991) 'Youth and AIDS in Russia', paper presented at 3rd International Symposium on AIDS Information and Education, Manila, Philippines, 3–7 February.

Chambers, R. (1997) *Whose Reality Counts? Putting the first last*, London: Intermediate Technology.

Chandhoke N. (2002) 'The Limits of Global Civil Society', in M. Glasius, M. Kaldor and H. Anheier (eds) *Global Civil Society 2002*, Oxford: Oxford University Press.

Chandler, D. (1998) 'Democratization in Bosnia: the Limits of Civil Society Building Strategies', *Democratization*, 5(4): 78–102.
—— (2005) *Constructing Global Civil Society. Morality and Power in International Relations*, New York: Palgrave McMillan.
Charachidzé, G. (1989) *Face aux drapeaux. Le genre humain*, Paris: Le Seuil.
Chauveau, J.-P., Jul-Larsen, E. and Chaboud, C. (eds) (2000) *Les pêches piroguières en Afrique de l'Ouest. Pouvoirs, mobilités, marchés*, Paris: CMI / IRD / Karthala.
Chervyakov, V. *et al.* (1998) 'Adolescent Sexuality in Russia', paper presented at 2nd Conference on Social Sciences and AIDS in Europe, Paris [AbSraC Sy 8.1].
Chouvy, P. A. (2002) *Les territoires de l'opium. Conflits et trafics du Triangle d'Or et du Croissant d'Or*, Genève: Olizane.
—— (2006) 'Afghanistan's Opium Production in Perspective', *China and Eurasia Forum Quarterly*, 4(1): 21–24.
Christenson G. A. (1997) 'World Civil Society and the International Rule of Law', *Human Rights Quarterly*, 19: 724–37.
Chuvin, P. (ed.) (2004) *Asie centrale, Annales. Histoire, sciences sociales*, Paris: EHESS.
Chuvin, P. and Gentelle, P. (1998) *L'Asie centrale entre communisme et intégrisme*, Paris: Marabout.
Clayton A. (ed.) (1997a) *Governance, Democracy and Conditionality: what Role for NGOs?*, Oxford: INTRAC Publications.
—— (1997b) *NGOs Civil Society and the State: Building Democracies in Transitional Countries*, Oxford: INTRAC Publications.
Colas, D. (1992) *Le glaive et le fléau. Généalogie du fanatisme et de la société civile*, Paris: Grasset.
Conquest, R. (1986) *The Harvest of Sorrow. Soviet Collectivization and the Terror-Famine*, New York: Oxford University Press.
Copans J. (2006) *Développement mondial et mutations des sociétés contemporaines*, Paris: Armand Colin.
Cornell, S. E. (2006) 'The Narcotics Threat in Greater Central Asia: From Crime-Terror Nexus to State Infiltration?', *China and Eurasia Forum Quarterly*, 4(1): 37–67.
Cornell, S. E. and Spector, R. A. (2001) 'Central Asia: More than Islamic Extremists', *The Washington Quarterly*, 25(1): 193–206.
Cornell, S. E. and Swanström, N. L. P. (2006) 'The Eurasian Drug Trade: A Challenge to Regional Security', *Problems of Post-Communism*, 53: 4.
Crewe, E. and Harrison, E. (1998) *Whose Development? An Ethnography of Aid*, London: Zed Books.
Critchlow, J. (1991) *Nationalism in Uzbekistan: A Soviet Republic's Road to Sovereignty*, Boulder, CO: Westview Press.
Danziger, R. (1996) 'An Overview of HIV Prevention in Central and Eastern Europe', *AIDSCare*, 8(6): 701–7.
Davidova, A., Bogoyavlensky, G., Volkova, N. *et al.* (1998) 'Drug Use and Potential Risk of HIV Infection in Russian Young People', paper presented at 2nd Conference on Social Sciences and AIDS in Europe, Paris.
Davies, C. M. (1983) 'The Economics of the Soviet Health System', in *The Soviet Economy in the 1980s: Problems and Prospects*, Washington DC: JEC / US Congress.
—— (1984) *The Health and Pharmaceutical Sectors of the Soviet Economy*, London: Wharton Econometric Forecasting Associates.

—— (1987) 'Development in the Health Sector of the Soviet Economy, 1970–90', in *Gorbachev's Economic Plans*, Vol. II, Washington DC: JEC / US Congress.
—— (1988) 'The Organization and Performance of the Contemporary Soviet Health Service', in G. W. Lapidus and G. E. Swanson (eds) *State and Welfare USA/USSR: Contemporary Policy and Practice*, Berkeley, CA: Institute of International Studies.
—— (1989) 'The Soviet Health System: a National Health Service in a Socialist Society', in M. G. Field (ed.) *Success and Crisis in National Health Systems: A Comparative Approach*, London: Routledge.
—— (1990) 'National Health Services, Resources Constraints and Shortages: a Comparison of Soviet and British Experiences', in N. Manning and C. Ungerson (eds) *Social Policy Review 1989–1990*, Harrow: Longman.
—— (1993) 'The Health Sector in the Soviet and Russian Economies: from Reform to Fragmentation to Transition', in *The Former Soviet Union in Transition*, vol. II, Washington DC: JEC / US Congress.
Davies, P., Hickson, F., Hunat, A., Weatherburn, P. and Project Sigma (1993) *Sex, Gay Men and AIDS*, London: Falmer Press.
Dawisha, K, and Parrott, B. (1994) *Russia and the New States of Eurasia. The Politics of Upheaval*, Cambridge: Cambridge University Press.
—— (eds) (1997) *Conflict, Cleavage and Change in Central Asia and the Caucasus*, New York: Cambridge University Press.
Dehne, K., Pokrovsky, V., Kobychscha, Y., Schwartländer, B. (2000) 'Update on the epidemics of HIV and other sexually transmitted infections in the newly independent states of the former Soviet Union', *AIDS*, 14: S75–84.
De Jong, B. (1982) '"An Intolerable Kind of Moral Degeneration": Homosexuality in the Soviet Union', *Review of Socialist Law*, 4: 341–57.
De Jong, W. M. (1996) 'HIV and Injecting Drug Use in Belarus, Svetlogorsk', UNAIDS report: unpublished.
—— (1997) 'HIV/AIDS Prevention in Odessa', UNAIDS report: unpublished.
Deler, J.-P., Faure, Y.-A., Piveteau, A. and Roca, P.-J. (1998) *ONG et développement. Société, économie, politique*, Paris: Karthala.
de Martino, L. (2005) 'La Suisse et l'Asie centrale: un processus d'apprentissage mutuel?', *Cemoti*, 36.
Demir, C. E., Balci, A. and Akkok, F. (2000) 'The Role of Turkish Schools in the Educational System and Social Transformation of Central Asian Countries: the case of Turkmenistan and Kyrgyztan', *Central Asian Survey*, 19(1): 141–56.
Des Jarlais, D. C., Grund, J.-P., Zadoretzky, C., Milliken, J., Friedmann, P., Titus, S., Perlis, T., Bodrova, V. and Zemlianova, E. (2002) 'HIV risk behaviour among participants of syringe exchange programmes in central/eastern Europe and Russia', *International Journal of Drug Policy*, 13: 165–70.
de Tocqueville, A. (1851) *Democracy in America, The Republic of the United States and Its Political Institutions*, Henry Reeves, translator, Garden City, NY: A.S. Barnes and Co.
Dhawan, S. and Narula, R. (1992) *Silent Killer*, New Delhi: First City.
Djalili, M. R.and Kellner, T. (2001) *Géopolitique de la nouvelle Asie centrale*, Paris: PUF.
Dowsett, G. W. (1996) *Practicing Desire: Homosexual Sex in the Era of AIDS*, Stanford, CT: Stanford University Press.
Dozon, J.-P. and Vidal, L. (eds) (1995) *Les sciences sociales face au SIDA*, Paris, ORSTOM Editions.

Earle, L. (2004) *Community Development in Kazakhstan, Kyrgyzstan and Uzbekistan: Lessons Learnt from Recent Experience*, Oxford: INTRAC Publications.

—— (2005) 'Community development, 'tradition' and the civil society strengthening agenda in Central Asia', *Central Asian Survey*, 24(3): 245–60.

Edward, M. and Hulme, D. (1996) 'Too Close for Comfort? The Impact of Official Aid on Nongovernmental Organizations', *World Development*, 24(6): 961–73.

Edwards, M. (2001) 'Introduction', in M. Edwards and J. Gaventa (eds) *Global Citizen Action*, London: Earthscan.

Elleinstein, J. (1992) *D'une Russie à l'autre: vie et mort de l'URSS*, Paris: Messidor.

Engelstein, L. (1992) *The Keys to Happiness: Sex and the Search for Modernity in Fin-de-Siècle Russia*, Ithaca, NY: Cornell University Press.

Escobar, A. (1991) 'Anthropology and the Development Encounter: the Making and Marketing of Development Anthropology', *American Ethnologist*, 18(4): 658–82.

—— (1996) *Encountering Development: the Making and Unmaking of the Third World*, Princeton, NJ: Princeton University Press.

EuroHIV (2005) *HIV/AIDS Surveillance in Europe: End-year report 2004*, No. 71. Institut de Veille Sanitaire de Saint-Maurice, report.

Everett-Heath, T. (ed.) (2003) *Central Asia. Aspects of Transition*, London: Routledge-Curzon.

Farmer, P. (1992) *AIDS and Accusation. Haiti and the Geography of Blame*, Berkeley, CA: University of California Press.

—— (1999a) *Infections and Inequalities. The Modern Plagues*, Berkeley, CA: University of California Press.

—— (1999b) *The Global Impact of Drug-Resistant Tuberculosis*, Cambridge, MA: Harvard Medical School and Open Society Institute.

—— (2003) *Pathologies of Power*, Berkeley, CA: University of California Press.

Farmer, P., Connors, M. and Simmons, J. (eds) (1996) *Women, Poverty and AIDS: Sex, Drugs and Structural Violence,* Monroe, ME: Common Courage.

Farmer, P., Lindenbaum, S. and Delvecchio-Good, M. J. (1993) 'Women, poverty and AIDS: an introduction', *Culture, Medicine and Psychiatry*, 17(4): 387–97.

Fassin, D. (1992) *Pouvoir et maladie en Afrique*, Paris: PUF, Les Champs de la Santé.

—— (1994) 'Le domaine privé de la santé publique. Pouvoir, politique et sida au Congo', *Annales, Histoire, Sciences Sociales*, 4: 745–75.

—— (1996) 'Idéologie, pouvoir et maladie. Eléments d'une anthropologie politique du sida en Afrique', in M. Cros (ed.), *Les maux de l'autre*, Paris: L'Harmattan, 65–94.

—— (2002) 'Embodied history. Uniqueness and exemplarity of South African Aids', *African Journal of Aids Research*, 1(1): 63–68.

—— (2004) *Afflictions. L'Afrique du Sud de l'apartheid au SIDA*, Paris: Karthala.

—— (2005) *When Bodies Remember. Experiences and Politics of AIDS in South Africa*, Berkeley, CA: University of California Press.

—— (2006) *Quand les corps se souviennent. Expériences et politiques du Sida en Afrique du Sud*, Paris: La découverte.

—— (2007) *When Bodies Remember: Experiences and Politics of AIDS in South Africa*, Berkeley, CA: University of California Press.

Fassin, D. and Rechtman, R. (2007) *L'empire du traumatisme. Enquête sur la condition de victime*, Paris: Flammarion. English translation in press, to be published by Princeton University Press.

Fassin, D. and Vasquez, P. (2005) 'Humanitarian exception as the rule: the political theology of the 1999 Tragedia in Venezuela', *American Ethnologist*, 32(3), 389–405.

Favarel-Garigues, G. (2003) *Criminalité, police et gouvernement: trajectoires post-communistes*, Paris: L'Harmattan.

Fenopetov, V. (2006) 'The Drug Crime Threat to Countries Located on the "Silk Road"', *China and Eurasia Forum Quarterly*, 4(1): 5–13.

Ferguson, J. (1990) *The Anti-Politics Machine: Development, Depolitization and Bureaucratic Powerin Lesotho*, Cambridge: Cambridge University Press.

—— (1997) 'Anthropology and its evil twin: development in the constitution of a discipline', in F. Cooper and R. Packard (eds) *International Development and the Social Sciences*, Berkeley, CA: University of California Press.

—— (1999) *Expectations of Modernity: Myths and Meanings of Urban Life on the Zambian Copperbelt*, Berkeley, CA: University of California Press.

Ferro, M. (1993) 'Après l'URSS, ruptures et continuités', in M. Ferro and M.-H. Mandrillon (eds) *L'état de toutes les Russies. Les États et les Nations de l'ex-URSS*, Paris: La Découverte / IMSECO.

—— (1999a) 'Nazisme et communisme: les limites d'une comparaison', in M. Ferro (ed.) *Nazisme et communisme: deux régimes dans le siècle*, Paris: Pluriel.

—— (1999b) 'Y a-t-il "trop de démocratie" en URSS?', in M. Ferro (ed.) *Nazisme et communisme: deux régimes dans le siècle*, Paris: Pluriel.

Ferro, M. and Mandrillon, M.-H. (eds) (1993) *L'état de toutes les Russies. Les États et les nations de l'ex-URSS*, Paris: La Découverte / IMSECO.

Field, M. (1957) *Doctor and Patient in Soviet Russia*, Cambridge, MA: Harvard University Press.

—— (1976) *Soviet Socialised Medicine: an Introduction*, New York: Free Press.

Field, M. G. (2004) 'HIV and AIDS in the Former Soviet Bloc', *New England Journal of Medicine*, 315: 117–20.

Flowers, R. (1991) 'On Being Queer in the USSR', *Metroline*, 12 (July): 12–13.

Foucault, M. (1965) *Madness and Civilization*, New York: Pantheon.

—— (1970) *The Order of Things*, New York: Pantheon.

—— (1972) *The Archaeology of Knowledge*, New York: Pantheon.

—— (1973) *Birth of the Clinic*, New York: Pantheon.

—— (1977) *Discipline and Punish*, New York: Pantheon.

—— (1978) *The History of Sexuality, Vol. I: An Introduction*, New York: Pantheon.

—— (1985) *The History of Sexuality, Vol. II: The Use of Pleasure*, New York: Random House.

—— (1986) *The History of Sexuality Vol. III: The Care of the Self*, New York: Random House.

Fourniau, V. (1994) *Histoire de l'Asie centrale*, Paris: PUF.

Freizer, S. (2005) 'Neo-liberal and communal civil society in Tajikistan: merging or dividing in the post-war period?', *Central Asian Survey*, 24(3): 225–43.

Garbutt, A. and Heap, S. (2003) *Growing Civil Society in Central Asia*, Oxford: INTRAC Publications, OPS 39.

Gardner, K. and Lewis, D. (1996) *Anthropology, Development and the Post-Modern Challenge*, London: Pluto Press.

Gardner, K. and Lewis, D. (2000) 'Dominant paradigms overturned or "business as usual"? Development discourse and the White Paper on International Development', *Critique of Anthropology*, 20(1): 15–29.

Geiss, P. G. (2006) 'State and Regime Change in central Asia', in A. Berg and A. Kreikemeyer (eds) *Realities of Transformation. Democratization Policies in Central Asia Revisited*, Baden-Baden: Nomos.

Gessen, M. (1994) *The Rights of Lesbians and Gay Men in the Russian Federation*, San Francisco, CA: International Gay and Lesbian Human Rights Commission.

Giffen, J., Earle, L. and Buxton, C. (2005) *The Development of Civil Society in Central Asia*, Oxford: INTRAC Publications, NGOMPS 17.

Gleason, G. (1998) *The Central Asian States*, Boulder, CO: Westview Press.

Godinho, J., Novotny, T., Tadesse, H. and Vinokur, A. (2004) *HIV/AIDS and Tuberculosis in Central Asia: Country Profiles*, Washington, DC: World Bank.

—— (2005) *Reversing the tide: priorities for HIV/AIDS prevention in Central Asia*, Washington, DC: World Bank.

Goldman, W. Z. (1993) *Women, the State and the Revolution. Soviet Family Policy and Social Life, 1917–1936*, Cambridge: Cambridge University Press.

Goodhand, J. (2000) 'From Holy War to Opium War? A Case Study of the Opium Economy in North Eastern Afghanistan', *Central Asian Survey*, 19(2): 265–80.

Goodwin, R., Kozlova, A., Kwiatkowska, A., Anh Nguyen Luu, L., Nizharadza, G., Realo, A., Kulvet, A. and Rammer, A. (2003) 'Social Representation of HIV/AIDS in Central and Eastern Europe', *Social Sciences and Medicine*, 56: 1373–84.

Goskomstat SSSR (1991) 'Spolzovaniye kontratseptsiy v SSR' Vestnik Satistiki, No. 3, 60, cited in A. Popov, A. P. Visser and E. Ketting, 'Contraceptive Knowledge, Attitudes and Practice in Russia during the 1980s', *Studies in Family Planning*, 24(4): 227–35.

Grillo, R. D. and Stirrat, R. L. (eds) (1997) *Discourses of Development. Anthropological Perspectives*, Oxford: Berg.

Grugel, J. (2003) 'Democratisation Studies Globalisation: The Coming of Age of a Paradigm', *British Journal of Politics and International Relations*, 5(2): 258–83.

Grund, J. P. (1996) 'Developing a Pragmatic Public Health Response to Drug Related Harm in Eastern Europe', Report, Lindshmit Center / Open Society Institute: unpublished.

Gunder, Frank A. (1992) 'The Development of Underdevelopment', in C. K. Wilber and K. P. Jameson (eds) *The Political Economy of Development and Underdevelopment*, 5th edition, New York: McGraw Hill.

Gupta, A. (1998) *Postcolonial Developments: Agriculture in the making of modern India,* Durham, NC: Duke University Press.

Gupta, A. and Ferguson, J. (eds) (1997) *Culture, Power, Place: Explorations in Critical Anthropology*, Durham, NC: Duke University Press.

Hann, C. M. (ed.) (2002a) *Postsocialism. Ideals, ideologies and practices in Eurasia*, London: Routledge.

—— (2002b) 'Postsocialism as a topic of anthropological investigation – Farewell to the socialist "other"', in C. M. Hann (ed.) *Postsocialism. Ideals, ideologies and practices in Eurasia*, London: Routledge.

Hann, C. M. and Dunn, E. (1996) *Civil Society. Challenging Western Models*, New York: Routledge.

Hamers, F. (1997) 'Monograph on HIV Infection in Ukraine', report, UNAIDS.

—— (2000) 'HIV infection in Ukraine (1987–96)', *Revue d'Epidémiologie et de Santé Publique* 48 (sup. 1): S3–15.

Hamers, F. and Downs, A. M. (2003) 'HIV in central and eastern Europe', *The Lancet* online review, 18 February 2003, available at http://image.thelancet.com/extras/02art6024web.pdf (retrieved 17 May 2005).

Harris, C. (1998) 'Coping with daily life in post-Soviet Tajikistan: the Gharmi villages of Khatlon province', *Central Asian Survey*, 17(4): 655–72.

Harrison, N. (2000) *Constructing Sustainable Development*, New York: State University of New York Press.

Healy, J. and Mckee, M. (1997) 'Health Sector Reform in Central and Eastern Europe: the Professional Dimension', *Health Policy and Planning*, 12(4): 286–95.

Heap, (2000) *NGOs Engaging with Business; A World of Difference and a Difference to the World*, Oxford: INTRAC Publications, OPS 33.

Heradstveit, D. (2001) 'Democratic development in Azerbaijan and the role of the Western oil industry', *Central Asian Survey*, 20(3): 261–88.

Hobart, M. (ed.) (1993) *An Anthropological Critique of Development: the Growth of Ignorance*, London: Routledge.

Hohman, S. (2004) 'Santé publique en Ouzbékistan contemporain: continuités soviétiques et limites des processus engagés', *Les Cahiers d'Asie Centrale* 13–14: 121–61.

Hohman, S. and Garenne, M. (2005) 'Vulnérabilité et santé en Ouzbékistan: analyse des différentiels de mortalité en fonction des richesses des ménages', *Annales de démographie historique* 2: 109–38.

Hours, B. (1998) *L'idéologie humanitaire ou le spectacle de l'altérité perdue*, Paris: L'Harmattan.

Howell, J. (1996) 'Poverty and transition in Kyrgyzstan: how some households cope', *Central Asia Survey*, 15(1): 59–73.

Hudock, A. C. (1999) *NGOs and Civil Society; Democracy by Proxy?*, Cambridge: Cambridge University Press.

Humes, D. and Edward, M. (1997) *NGOs, States and Donors, Too Close for Comfort?*, New York: Save the Children Press.

Hunt, M. (2001) *"Top-down-Bottom-up"? A Study of Women's Participation in NGOs in Kyrgyzstan*, Oxford: INTRAC Publications, OPS 34.

Hunter, S. (2003) *AIDS in Africa*, New York: Macmillan.

—— (2005) *AIDS in Asia*, New York: St. Martins Press.

Hyde, G. (1974) *The Soviet Health Service: a Historical and Comparative Study*, London: Lawrence and Wishart.

Hyman, A. (1994) *Political Change in post-Soviet Central Asia*, London: Post-Soviet Business Forum / Royal Institute of International Affairs.

Ilkhamov, A. (2005) 'The thorny path of civil society in Uzbekistan', *Central Asian Survey*, 24(3): 297–317.

Ingram, M. (1997) 'Russia Fears Rapid Increase of HIV Infection', *British Medical Journal*, 314: 1783.

International Center for Non-Profit Law (1998) 'NGO Legislation and its Implementation in Central Asia', report: unpublished.

International Crisis Group (2001) 'Central Asia: Drugs and Conflict', report: unpublished.

International Labour Organization (1976) *Employment, Growth and Basic Needs: a One World Problem*, Geneva: ILO Press.

Jackson, N. (2005) 'The Trafficking of Narcotics, Arms and Humans in post-Soviet Central Asia: (Mis)perceptions, Policies and Realities', *Central Asian Survey*, 24(1): 39–52.

James, R. (ed.) (2001) *Power and Partnership? Experience of NGO Capacity Building*, Oxford: INTRAC Publications.

—— (ed.) (2005) *Building Organisational Resilience to HIV/AIDS: Implications for Capacity Building*, Oxford: INTRAC Publications, Praxis Paper 4.

Kaldor, M. (2003) *Global Civil Society: An Answer to War*, Cambridge: Polity Press.
Kalibala, S., Rubaramira, R. and Kaleeba, N. (1997) 'Non-Governmental Organizations and Community Responses to HIV/AIDS and the Role of HIV-Positive Persons in Prevention and Care', *AIDS*, 11 (sup. B): 5151–57.
Kalinin, S. (1990) 'Letter from Leningrad', *Gay Times*, August: 38–40.
Kandiyoti, D. (1996) 'Modernization without the market? The case of the Soviet East', *Economy and Society*, 25(4): 529–42.
—— (1998) 'Rural livelihoods and social networks in Uzbekistan: perspectives from Andijan', *Central Asian Survey* 17(4): 561–78.
—— (2002) *Agrarian Reform, Gender and Land Rights in Uzbekistan*, Geneva: UNRISD.
—— (2004) *Post Soviet Institutional Design, NGOs and Rural Livelihoods in Uzbekistan, Civil Society and Social Movements (2000–2205)*, Programme Paper 11, Geneva: UNRISD.
Kandiyoti, D. and Mandel, R. (1998) 'Editors' preface', *Central Asian Survey*, 17(4): 533–37.
Kaser, M. (1976) *Health Care in the Soviet Union and Eastern Europe*, London: Croom Helm.
—— (1997) 'Economic transition in six Central Asian economies', *Central Asian Survey*, 16(1): 5–26.
Katoff, L. and Ince, S. (1991) 'Supporting People with AIDS: the GMHC Model', in N. F. McKenzie and G. A. Lloyd (eds) *The AIDS Reader*, New York: Meridian.
Kazakhstan AIDS Centre (2001) *Behavioural Survey among Injecting Drug Users in Nine Cities of Kazakhstan*, Almaty: Republican AIDS Centre.
—— (2004) *Results of 2003 Sentinel Epidemiological Surveillance for HIV among Sex Workers in Kazakhstan*, Almaty: Republican AIDS Centre.
—— (2005) *HIV/AIDS in Kazakhstan*, fact sheet.
Kendall, C. (1991) 'Commentary on epidemiologists, social scientists and the structure of medical research on AIDS in Africa', *Social Science and Medicine*, 33(7): 785–86.
—— (1995) 'The Construction of Risk in AIDS Control Programs: Theoretical Bases and Popular Responses', in R. Parker and J. Gagnon, (eds) *Conceiving Sexuality: Approaches to Sex Research in a Postmodern World*, New York: Routledge.
—— (2005) 'Waste not, want not: penny capitalism and global lessons for water use from Lima, Peru' in L. Whiteford and S. Whiteford (eds) *New Advances in Water and Anthropology*, Santa Fe, NM: School of American Research Press.
Khodakevich, L., Kobyscha, Y., Shcherbinskaya, A. M. *et al.* (1997) 'Development of HIV Epidemic in Belarus, Moldova and Ukraine', paper presented at the 8th International Conference on the Reduction of Drug Related Harm, Paris, March.
Knaus, W. (1982) *Inside Russian Medicine*, New York: Everest House.
Kobysha, Y., Shcherbinskaya, A. M., Khodakevich, L., Andrushchak, L. and Kon, I. (1989) *Psikhologiya rannei yunost*, Moscow: Prosveshchenie.
—— (1991) *Vkus zapretnovo ploda*, Moscow: Molodaya gvardia.
—— (1992) 'Culture and Sexuality in the Former USSR', *Planned Parenthood in Europe*, 21(2): 2–4.
—— (1995) *The Sexual Revolution in Russia*, New York: The Free Press.
Kon, I. and Riordan, J. (eds) (1993) *Sex and Russian Society*, London: Pluto Press.
Konings, E. (1996) 'Prostitution and HIV/AIDS in CEE/CIS', UNAIDS report: unpublished.

Kosukhin, A. B. (1998) 'Epidemiological Situation with Regard to Sexually Transmitted Diseases and Introduction of Modern Treatment and Monitoring Methods among Patients in the Kyrgyz Republic', UNDP report: unpublished.

Kramer, L. (1988) *The Beginning of Acting Up*, New York: St. Martins Press.

Kruglov, Y. (1996) 'HIV Infection among Drug Users in the Ukraine: Beginning of the Epidemic', paper presented at the 8th International Conference on AIDS, Vancouver, July.

Kuehnast, K. (1998) 'From pioneers to entrepreneurs: young women, consumerism, and the "world picture" in Kyrgyzstan', *Central Asian Survey*, 17(4): 639–54.

Kulchik, Y., Fadin, A. and Sergeev, V. (1996) *Central Asia after the Empire*, London: Pluto Press.

Kurova, T., Shoubnikova, M., Malceva, A. and Mardh, P. A. (1998) 'Prostitution in Riga, Latvia. A Socio-Medical Matter of Concern', *Acta Obset Gynecol Scand*, 77(1): 83–86.

Lachapelle, G. and Paquin, S. (eds) (2004) *Mondialisation, gouvernance et nouvelles stratégies subétatiques*, Québec: Presses de l'Université Laval.

Laplantine, F. (2003) *De tout petits liens*, Paris : Mille et Une Nuits.

Laroche, J. (ed.) (2003) *Mondialisation et gouvernance mondiale*, Paris: PUF.

Larrain, J. (1989) *Theories of Development. Capitalism, Colonialism and Dependency*, Cambridge: Polity Press.

Laruelle, M. (2004) 'Mondialisation et altermondialisme dans les réflexions des milieux politiques et intellectuels d'Asie centrale', *La Pensée*, 338: 27–36.

Laruelle, M. and Peyrouse, S. (2006) *Asie centrale, la dérive autoritaire*, Paris: Autrement.

Latour, B. (1987) *Science in Action, How to Follow Scientists and Engineers through Society*, Cambridge, MA: Harvard University Press.

—— (1993) *We have never been modern* (English translation revised and augmented), Cambridge, MA: Harvard University Press.

—— (1999) *Pandora's Hope. Essays on the Reality of Science Studies*, Cambridge, MA: Harvard University Press.

Lautier, B. (1994) *L'économie informelle dans le Tiers Monde*, Paris: La Découverte / IMSECO.

—— (2001) 'Sous la morale, la politique. La Banque mondiale et la lutte contre la pauvreté', *Politique africaine*, 82: 169–76.

Ledeneva, A. (1998) *Russia's Economy of Favours*, Cambridge: Cambridge University Press.

Lester, D. (1999) 'Suicide in post-Soviet Central Asia', *Central Asian Survey*, 18(1): 121–24.

Levitin, L. (2001) *Uzbekistan on an historical threshold?*, Chesterton, UK: Granta Editions.

Liitsola, K., Tashkinova, I., Laukkanen, T. *et al.* (1998) 'HIV-1 Genetic Subtype a/b Recombinant Strain Causing an Explosive Epidemic in Injecting Drug Users in Kaliningrad', *AIDS*, 12: 1907–19.

Lindenbaum, S. and Lock, M. (1993) *Knowledge and Practice. The Anthropology of Medicine and Everyday Life*, Berkeley, CA: University of California Press.

Linglof, T. (1995) 'Rapid Increase of Syphilis and Gonorrhoea in Parts of the Former USSR', *Sexually Transmitted Diseases*, 22(3): 160–61.

Lisitsyn, Y. (1972) *Health Protection in the USSR*, Moscow: Progress.

Lock, M. and Scheper-Hughes, N. (1996) 'A Critical-Interpretative Approach in Medical Anthropology: Rituals and Routine of Discipline and Dissent', in C. Sargent and T. M. Johnson (eds) *Medical Anthropology*, Westport, CT: Praeger.

Long, N. (2001) *Sociology of Development: Actors' perspectives*, London: Routledge.

Long, N. and Long, A. (1992) *Battlefields of Knowledge: the Interlocking of Theory and Practice in Social Research and Development*, London: Routledge.

Lowndes, C. M., Alary, M. and Platt, L. (2003) 'Editorial: Injection Drug Use, Commercial Sex Work, and the HIV/STI Epidemic in the Russian Federation', *Sexually Transmitted Diseases*, 30(1): 46–48.

Lunin, I., Hall, T. H., Mandel, J. S. *et al.* (1995) 'Adolescent Sexuality in St. Petersburg, Russia', *AIDS*, 9(1): S53–S60.

Luong-Jones, P. (2002) Institutional change and continuity in post-Soviet Central Asia, New York: Cambridge University Press.

—— (ed.) (2004) The Transformation of Central Asia: States and Societies from Soviet rule to independence, Ithaca, NY: Cornell University Press.

Luong-Jones, P. and Weinthal, E. (1999) 'The NGO paradox: democratic goals and non-democratic outcomes in Kazakhstan', *Europe-Asia Studies*, 51(7): 1267–84.

Maina, W. (1998) 'Kenya: The State, Donors and the Politics of democratization', in van Rooy (ed.) *Civil Society and the Aid Industry*, London: Earthscan.

Makarenko, T. (2002) 'Crime, Terror, and the Central Asian Drug Trade', *Harvard Asia Quarterly*, 6: 3.

Malinowska-Sempruch, K. (2002) 'Barcelona 2002: law, ethics, and human rights. The need for harm-reduction approaches in Eastern Europe and the former Soviet Union', *Canadian HIV AIDS Policy Law Review*, 7(2–3): 84–88.

Malinowska-Sempruch, K. and Gallagher, S. (eds) (2004) *War on Drugs, HIV/Aids and Human Rights*, Sourcebook on Contemporary Controversies, New York: Idea Press.

Malkki, L. (1995) *Purity and Exile: Violence, Memory, and National Cosmology among Hutu Refugees in Tanzania*, Chicago, IL: Chicago University Press.

Mandel, R. (2002) 'Seeding civil society', in C. E. Hann (ed.) *Postsocialism. Ideals, ideologies and practices in Eurasia*, London: Routledge.

Mandelbaum, M. (ed.) (1994) *Central Asia. Kazakhstan, Uzbekistan, Tajikistan, Kyrgyzstan, Turkmenistan andthe World*, New York: Council on Foreign Relations Press.

Mandrillon, M.-H. (1992) 'La conquête du pouvoir local en Russie', in *Problèmes politiques et sociaux*, Paris: La Documentation française.

—— (1993) 'Des hommes de l'ancien régime', in M. Ferro and M.-H. Mandrillon (eds) *L'état de toutes les Russies. Les États et les nations de l'ex-URSS*, Paris: La Découverte / IMSECO.

Mann, J. M., Tarantola, D. J. M. and Netter, T. W. (eds) (1995) *AIDS in the World*, Cambridge, MA: Harvard University Press.

Marcus, G. (1995) 'Ethnography in/of the world system: the emergence of multi-sited ethnography', *Annual Review of Anthropology*, 24: 95–117.

Marcus, M. (1998) *Ethnography through thick and thin*, Princeton, NJ: Princeton University Press.

Marie, A. (2005) *La coopération décentralisée et ses paradoxes: dérives bureaucratiques et notabiliaires du développement local en Afrique*, Paris: Karthala.

Massicard, E. and Trevisani, T. (2003) 'The Uzbek Mahalla. Between State and Society' in T. Everett-Heath (ed.) *Central Asia. Aspects of Transition*, London: Routledge-Curzon.

Matic, S., Lazarus, J. V. and Donoghoe, M. C. (eds) (2006) *HIV/AIDS in Europe: Moving from death sentence to chronic disease management*, Geneva: WHO.

Mawdsley, E., Townsend, J., Porter, G. and Oakley, P. (2002) *Knowledge, Power and Development Agenda: NGOs North and South*, Oxford: INTRAC Publications, NGOMPS 14.

Medvedev, Z. A. (1990) 'Evolution of AIDS policy in the Soviet Union: II – the AIDS epidemic and emergency measures', *British Medical Journal*, 7: 932–34.

Megoran, N. (2005) 'Preventing conflict by building civil society: post-development theory and a Central Asian – UK policy success story', *Central Asian Survey*, 24(1): 83–96.

Mehrotra, S. (1999) 'Public spending priorities and the poor in Central Asia', in *Central Asia 2010. Prospects for Human Development*, New York: UNDP.

Melvin, N. J. (2000) *Uzbekistan. Transition to Authoritarianism on the Silk Road*, Amsterdam: Harwood Academic Publishers.

Mendras, M. (1992) *Un État pour la Russie*, Bruxelles: Éditions Complexe.

Mikkelsen, H. (1996) 'Men Who Have Sex with Men in Former USSR', UNAIDS report: unpublished.

Miller, N. (1992) *Out of the World*, New York: Random House.

Moatti, J.-P. and Souterrand, Y. (2000) 'HIV/AIDS Social and Behavioural Research: Past Advances and Thoughts about the Future', *Social Sciences and Medicine*, 50: 1519–32.

Morris, M., Podhisita, C., Wawer, M. S. and Handcock, M. S. (1996) 'Bridge Populations in the Spread of HIV/AIDS in Thailand', *AIDS*, 10(11): 1265–71.

Mosse, D. (2005) *Cultivating Development: An Ethnography of Aid Policy and Practice*, London: Pluto Press.

Motyl, J. (ed.) (1992a) *The Post-Soviet Nations. Perspectives on the Demise of the USSR*, New York: Columbia University Press.

—— (1992b) *Thinking Theoretically about Soviet Nationalities*, New York: Columbia University Press.

—— (1992c) 'The End of Sovietology: from Soviet Studies to Post-Soviet Studies', in A. J. Motyl (ed.) *The Post-Soviet Nations. Perspectives on the Demise of the USSR*, New York: Columbia University Press.

—— (ed.) (1995) *Thinking Theoretically about Soviet Nationalities. History and Comparison in the Study of the USSR*, New York: Columbia University Press.

Muet, P. A. (1993) *Le développement*, Paris: La Documentation française / Conseil d'analyse économique.

National Statistics Committee of the Kyrgyz Republic (2000) *Kyrgyzstan in Figures*, Bishkek: National Statistics Committee of the Kyrgyz Republic.

Navarro, V. (1977) *Social Security and Medicine in the USSR: a Marxist Critique*, Lexington, MD: Lexington Books.

Olcott, M. B. (2002) *Kazakhstan: Unfulfilled Promise*, Washington, DC: Carnegie Endowment for International Peace.

Olivier de Sardan, J.-P. (1995) *Anthropologie et développement. Essai en socio-anthropologie du changement social*, Paris: Karthala.

—— (2002) 'Les trois approches en anthropologie du développement', *Tiers-Monde*, 168: 729–53.

Olivier de Sardan, J. P, Biershenk, T. and Chauveau J. P. (2000) *Courtiers en développement. Les villages africains en quête de projets*, Paris: Karthala.

Oostvogels, R. (1997) 'Assessment of Interventions among Men Who Have Sex with Men in Bishkek, Kyrgyzstan', WHO Bishkek, report: unpublished.

Oostvogels, R. and Mikkelsen, H. (1998) 'Assessment of the Situation Regarding HIV and Men Who Have Sex with Men in Tashkent, Uzbekistan', UNAIDS Tashkent, report: unpublished.

Osmont, A. (1998) 'La "gouvernance": concept mou, politique ferme', *Les Annales de la Recherche Urbaine*, 80–81: 19–26.

Paksoy, H. B. (1994) *Central Asia Reader. The Rediscovery of History*, Armonk, NY: M. E. Sharpe.

Pandolfi, M. (2003) 'Contract of Mutual (In)Difference: Governance and Humanitarian Apparatus in Albania and Kosovo', *Indiana Journal of Global Legal Studies*, 10(1): 369–81.

Parker, R. (1990) 'The Response to AIDS in Brazil', in B. Mitsztal and D. Moss (eds) *Action on AIDS*, New York: Greenwood Press.

—— (1996) 'Empowerment, Community Mobilization and Social Change in the Face of the HIV/AIDS', *AIDS*, 10 (sup. 3): S27–S31.

—— (1999) *Beneath the Equator: Cultures of desire, Male homosexuality and Emerging Gay Communities in Brazil*, New York: Routledge.

—— (2001) 'Sexuality, culture and power in HIV/AIDS research', *Annual Review of Anthropology*, 30: 163–79.

—— (2002) 'The Global HIV/AIDS pandemic, structural inequalities, and the politics of international health', *American Journal of Public Health*, 93(3): 343–46.

Parker, R. and Aggleton, P. (eds) (1999) *Culture, Society and Sexuality: A Reader*, London: UCL Press.

Parker, R., and Ehrhardt, A. A. (2001) 'Through an ethnographic lens: Ethnographic methods, comparative analysis, and HIV/AIDS research', *AIDS and Behavior*, 5(2):105–14.

Parker, R. and Gagnon, J. (eds) (1995) *Conceiving Sexuality: Approaches to Sex Research in Postmodern World*, New York: Routledge.

Parker, R. and Herbert, D. (1993) *Sexuality, Politics and AIDS in Brazil*, London: The Falmer Press.

Parker, R., Barbosa, R. M., Aggleton, P. (eds) (2000) *Framing the Sexual Subject: The Politics of Gender, Sexuality and Power*, Berkeley, CA: University of California Press.

Parker, R., Khan, S. and Aggleton, P. (1998) 'Conspicuous by their absence? Men who have sex with men (MSM) in developing countries – implications for intervention', *Critical Public Health*, 8(4): 329–46.

Peters, G. and Pierre, J. (1998) 'Governance without Government? Rethinking Public Administration', *Journal of Public Administration Research and Theory: J-PART*, 8(2) (April): 223–43.

Pétric, B. M. (2002) *Pouvoir, don, réseaux en Ouzbékisan post-soviétique*, Paris: PUF.

—— (2005) 'Post-Soviet Kyrgyzstan or the Birth of a Globalized Protectorate', *Central Asian Survey*, 24(3):319–32.

Peyrouse, S. (ed.) (2005) *Gestion de l'indépendance et legs soviétique en Asie centrale*, in *Cahiers d'Asie centrale*, Nos 13–13. Paris: IFEAC / Edisud.

Pokrovskii, V., Federal AIDS Centre, 2005, 'HIV/AIDS in Russia', Presentation on HIV/AIDS at the Russian Federation and Ukraine workshop, Geneva, January.

Pokrovskii, V. V., Eramova, I. I., Deulina, M. *et al.* (1990) 'An intrahospital outbreak of HIV infection in Elista' (in Russian), *Zh Mikrobiol Epidemiol Immunobiol*, 4: 17–23.

Popovsky, M. (1983) *Trety Lishny: On, Ona i Sovietski Rezhim*, London: Overseas Publications.

Pottier, J. (1997) 'Towards an Ethnography of Participatory Appraisal', in R. D. Grillo and J. Stirrat (eds) *Discourses of Development: Anthropological Perspectives*, Oxford: Berg.

Poujol, C. (ed.) (1992) *Asie centrale. Aux confins des Empires, réveil et tumulte*, Paris: Autrement.

—— (1993) 'L'Asie centrale', in M. Ferro and M.-H. Mandrillon (eds) *L'état de toutes les Russies. Les États et les nations de l'ex-URSS*, Paris: La Découverte / IMSECO.

—— (1997) 'Cosaques et Kazakhs: nationalismes, identités et territoire', *Hérodote, le cercle de Samarcande*, 84: 124–43.

—— (2000) *Le Kazakhstan*, Paris: PUF.

—— (2001a) *L'islam en Asie centrale: vers la nouvelle donne*, Paris: Ellipses.

—— (2001b) *Dictionnaire de l'Asie centrale*, Paris: Ellipses.

—— (2004) 'How we can use the concept of transition for central Asian Post-Soviet History, an attempt to set a new approach', in CIMEAR, *The illusions of Transition: which perspective for Central Asia and the Caucasus?*, Geneva: CIMEAR, pp. 7–19.

—— (2005) *Ouzbékistan. La croisée des chemins*, Paris: Belin / La documentation française.

Powell, D. E. (1998) 'The Dismal State of Health Care in Russia', *Current History*, 97(621) (October): 335.

Pratt, B. (ed.) (2003) *Changing Expectations? The Concept and Practice of Civil Society in International Development*, Oxford: INTRAC Publications, NGOMPS 16.

Prebisch, R. (1950) *The Economic Development of Latin America and Its Principal Problems*, New York: United Nations.

Quarles Van Ufford, P. and Giri, A. (2003) *A Moral Critique of Development. In Search of Global Responsibilities*, New York: EIDOS.

Raballand, G. (2005) *L'Asie centrale ou la fatalité de l'enclavement?* Paris: L'Harmattan / IFEAC.

Rabinow, P. (1977) *Reflections on Fieldwork in Morocco*, Berkeley, CA: University of California Press.

—— (1986) 'Representations are Social Facts: Modernity and Post-Modernity in Anthropology', in J. Clifford and G. Marcus (eds) *Writing Culture: The Poetics and Politics of Ethnography*, Berkeley, CA: Berkeley University Press.

Radvanyi, J. (1990) *L'URSS, Régions et Nations*, Paris: Masson.

—— (1993) 'Un territoire en redéfinition' in M. Ferro and M.-H. Mandrillon (eds) *L'état de toutes les Russies. Les États et les nations de l'ex-URSS*, Paris: La Découverte / IMSECO.

—— (1997) *De l'URSS à la CEI, 12 États en quête d'identité*, Paris: Ellipses.

—— (ed.) (2003) *Les Etats post-soviétiques. Identités en construction, transformations politiques, trajectoires économiques*, Paris: Armand Colin.

Rashid, A. (1994) *The Resurgence of Central Asia: Islam or Nationalism?*, Karachi: Oxford University Press / London: Zed Books.

Rasizade, A. (2002) 'Azerbaijan after a decade of independence: less oil, more graft and poverty', *Central Asian Survey*, 21(4): 349–70.

Rechel, B. and McKee, M. (2005) *Human rights and health in Turkmenistan*, London: London School of Hygiene and Tropical Medicine.

Redfield, P. (2005) 'Doctors, Borders and Life in Crisis', *Cultural Anthropology*, (20)3: 328–61.

Renton, A. M., Borisenko, K. K., Meheus, A. and Gramyko, A. (1998) 'Epidemic of Syphilis in the Newly Independent States of the Former Soviet Union', *Sexually Transmitted Infections*, 74(3): 165–66.

Rhodes, T., Stimson, G. V., Crofts, N., Ball, A., Dehne, K. and Khodakevich, L. (1999) 'Drug Injecting, Rapid HIV Spread, and the "Risk Environment" Implications for Assessment and Response', *AIDS*, 13(A): S259–69.

Rhodes, T., Ball, A., Stimson, G. V. *et al.* (1999) 'HIV infection associated with drug injecting in the Newly Independent States and Eastern Europe: the social and economic context of epidemics', *Addiction*, 94: 1323–36.

Ribeiro, G. L. and Escobar, A. (2006) *Systems of Power*, Oxford: Berg.

Rich, V. (1987) 'AIDS Arrives in Soviet Union – (Official)', *Nature*, 326(5): 3.

Riordan, J. (1990) 'Coming out: the Gay Community in the USSR', *Slovo*, 3(1): 51–66.

Robertson, A. F. (1984) *People and the State: An Anthropology of Planned Development*, New York: Cambridge University Press.

Robinson, M. (1993) 'Will Political Conditionality Work?', *IDS Bulletin*, 24: 58–65.

Romer, J.-C., de Tinguy, A. *et al.* (1992) *La fin d'un empire: de l'URSS à la CEI*, Paris: Observatoire de l'URSS et de la CEI-FEDN.

Rosenau, J. and Czempiel, E. O. (1992) *Governance without Government: Order and Change in World Politics*, Cambridge: Cambridge University Press.

Rostow, W. W. (1960) *The Stages of Economic Growth*, Cambridge: Cambridge University Press.

Roux, J.-P. (1997) *L'Asie centrale. Histoire et civilisations*, Paris: Fayard.

Roy, O. (1991) 'Ethnies et politique en Asie centrale', *Revue du monde musulman et de la Méditerranée*, vol: 59–60.

—— (1992) 'Frontières et ethnies en Asie centrale', *Hérodote*, 64: 169–82.

—— (1997) *La nouvelle Asie centrale, ou la fabrication des nations*, Paris: Le Seuil.

—— (1999) 'Kolkhoz and civil society in the independent states of Central Asia', in M. Holt Ruffin and Daniel C. Waugh (eds) *Civil Society in Central Asia*, Seattle: Center for Civil Society International and Washington University Press.

—— (2001) *L'Asie centrale contemporaine*, Paris: PUF.

—— (2002) 'Soviet legacies and Western Aid imperatives in the new Central Asia', in A. Sajoo (ed.) *Civil Society in the Muslim World: Contemporary Perspectives*, London: I.B. Tauris.

Ruffin, M. H. and Waugh, D. (1999) *Civil Society in Central Asia*, Seattle, WA: Center for Civil Society International and Washington University Press.

Rumer, B. (1989) *Soviet Central Asia. A Tragic Experiment*, Boston, MA: Unwin Hyman.

—— (ed.) (1996) *Central Asia in transition: Dilemmas of political and economic development*, London: M. E. Sharpe.

Rupnik, J. (1988) 'Totalitarianism Revisited', in J. Keane (ed.) *Civil Society and the State: New European Perspective*, London: Verso.

Ryan, T. M. (1978) *The Organisation of Soviet Medical Care*, London: Martin Robertson.

—— (1987) 'Funding for the Soviet Health Service', *British Medical Journal*, 12: 652–53.

—— (1991) 'Policy and Administration in the Soviet Health Service', *Social Policy and Administration*, 25(3): 227–337.

Ryfman, P. (2004) *Les ONG*, Paris: La Découverte.

Saar, A., Kaldmae, P., Sodor, K. and Vaabel, A. (1998) 'Drug Use and Risk Taking Behaviour among Estonian Adolescents', paper presented at the 2nd Conference on Social Sciences and AIDS in Europe, Paris, January.

Saillant, F. (2003) 'L'Humanitaire, le corps, la citoyenneté. Imaginaire universaliste, transnationalismes et métissages', Actes du colloque Brésil/Montréal, CELAT, UQAM.

Saillant, F., Richardson, M. and Paumier, M. (2005) 'L'humanitaire et les identités. Un regard anthropologique', *Ethnologies*, 27(2): 160–87.

Safonov, A. G. and Loginova, Y. A. (1976) *Osnovy organizatsii satsionarnoi promyshlennosi*, Moscow: Meditsina.

Salomon, L. M. (1994) 'The Rise of the Nonprofit Sector: A Global 'Associational Revolution'', *Foreign Affairs*, 73(4): 109–22.

Saltmarshe, D. (1996) 'Civil society and sustainable development in Central Asia', *Central Asian Survey*, 15(3/4): 387–99.

Sapir, J. (1993a) 'Les contours de l'après-guerre froide', in M. Ferro and M.-H. Mandrillon (eds) *L'état de toutes les Russies. Les États et les nations de l'ex-URSS*, Paris: La Découverte / IMESCO.

—— (1993b) 'Une crise économique qui vient de loin', in M. Ferro and M.-H. Mandrillon (eds) *L'état de toutes les Russies. Les États et les nations de l'ex-URSS*, Paris: La Découverte / IMESCO.

—— (1993c) *Feu le système soviétique? Permanences politiques et mirages économiques, enjeux stratégiques*, Paris: La Découverte.

Schluter, D. P. (2002) *Gay Life in the Former USSR*, New York: Routledge.

Schoeberlein, J. (1999) 'Central Asian Studies in an International Context', in B. Schlyter and M. Juntunen (eds) *Re-entering the Silk Routes: Current Scandinavian Research on Central Asia*, New York: Kegan Paul International.

—— (2000a) 'Shifting Ground: How the Soviet Regime Used Resettlement to Transform Central Asian Society and the Consequences of This Policy Today', in H. Komatsu, C. Obiya and J. Schoeberlein (eds) *Migration in Central Asia: Its History and Current Problems*, Osaka: Japan Centre for Area Studies.

—— (2000b) 'The Caspian Region: Geography, Population and National Identity', in A. Ilkhamov and H. Amirahmadi (eds) *The Caspian Region at a Crossroad: Challenges of a New Frontier of Energy and Development*, New York: St. Martin's Press.

—— (2000c) 'Between Two Worlds: Obstacles to Development and Prosperity', *Harvard International Review*, 22(1): 56–61.

—— (2002) 'Central Asia: A Host of Preventable Conflicts', in P. van Tongeren, H. van de Veen and J. Verhoeven (eds) *Searching for Peace in Europe and Eurasia: An Overview of Conflict Prevention and Peacebuilding Activities*, Boulder, CO: Lynne Rienner.

Schraeder, P. J. (ed.) (2002) *Exporting Democracy: Rhetoric vs. Reality*, Boulder, CO: Lynne Rienner.

Scoones, I. and Thompson, J. (1994) *Beyond Farmer First: Rural Peoples' Knowledge, Agricultural Research and Extension Practice* London: Intermediate Technology Publication.

Scott, J. (1985) *Weapons of the Weak: Everyday Forms of Peasant Resistance*, New Haven, CT: Yale University Press.

—— (1990) *Domination and the Arts of Resistance: Hidden Transcripts*, New Haven, CT: Yale University Press.

Seidel, G. and Vidal, L. (1997) 'The implications of 'medical', 'gender in development' and 'culturalist' discourses for HIV/AIDS policy in Africa', in C. Shore and S. Wright (eds), *Anthropology of policy. Critical perspectives on governance and power*, London: Routledge, pp.59–87.

Serenko, F. *et al.* (1976) *Osnovy organizatsii poliklinicheskoi pomoshchi naseleniia*, Moscow: Meditsina.

Shkolnikov, V., McKee, M. and Lean, D. A. (2001) 'Changes in Life Expectancy in Russia in the Mid-1990s', *The Lancet*, 357: 917–21.

Shlapentokh V. (1989) *Public and Private Life of the Soviet People*, New York: Oxford University Press.

Shore, C. and Wright, S. (1997) *Anthropology of Policy. Critical Perspective on Governance and Power*, London: Routledge.

Sievers, E. W. (2003) *The Post-Soviet Decline in Central Asia. Sustainable development and comprehensive capital*, London and New York: Routledge and Curzon.

Singer, M. (1994) 'AIDS and the health crisis of the US urban poor: the perspective of critical medical anthropology', *Social Science and Medicine*, 39: 931–48.

—— (ed.) (1998) *The Political Economy of AIDS*, Amityville, New York: Baywood.

Smouts, M.-C. (1998) 'Du bon usage de la gouvernance en relations internationales', *Revue internationaledes sciences sociales*, 155: 85–94.

Solow, R. (1993) 'Sustainability: an Economist's Perspective', in R. Dorfman and N. S. Dorfman (eds) *Economics of the Environment: Selected Readings*, New York: W. W. Norton & Company.

Soucek, S. (2000) *A History of Inner Asia*, Cambridge: Cambridge University Press.

Stevens, D. (2005) 'NGO-Mahalla partnerships: exploring the potential for state-society synergy in Uzbekistan', *Central Asian Survey*, 24(3): 281–96.

Stirrat, R. L. (1996) 'The New Orthodoxy and Old Truths: Participation, Empowerment and Other Buzz Words', in S. Bastian and N. Bastian (eds) *Assessing Participation: A Debate from South Asia*, Delhi: Konark Publishers.

—— (2000) 'Cultures of consultancy', *Critique of Anthropology*, 20(1): 31–46.

Stoker, G. (1998) 'Cinq propositions pour une théorie de la gouvernance', *Revue Internationale des Sciences Sociales*, 155: 19–30.

Strada, V. (1992) 'Fin d'un empire, naissance d'une nation', in M. Mendras (ed.) *Un État pour la Russie*, Bruxelles: Éditions Complexe.

Tichonova, L., Borisenko, K., Ward, H., Meheus, A., Gromyko, A. and Renton, A. (1997) 'Epidemics of Syphilis in the Russian Federation: Trends, Origins and Priorities for Control', *The Lancet*, 350(9072): 210–13.

Todd, C.S. *et al.* (2005) 'Human immunodeficiency virus (HIV) infection in female sex workers in Tashkent, Uzbekistan', paper presented at the 16th biennial meeting of the International Society for Sexually Transmitted Diseases Research, Amsterdam, 10–13 July.

Tolipov, F. (2006) 'Power, Nation-building and Legacy – A comparative Analysis of Central Asian Leadership', in A. Berg and A. Kreikemeyer (eds) *Realities of Transformation. Democratization Policies in Central Asia Revisited*, Baden-Baden: Nomos.

Townsend, J. (2006) 'The Logistics of Opiate Trafficking in Tajikistan, Kyrgyzstan and Kazakhstan', *China and Eurasia Forum Quarterly*, 4(1): 69–91.

UNAIDS, (1999a) 'Un-Facilitated Response to HIV/AIDS, STD and Drug Use in Central Asian Countries: Kazakhstan, Kyrgyzstan, Tajikistan, Turkmenistan, Uzbekistan, 1996–98', report.

—— (1999b) *L'ONUSIDA et les organisations non gouvernementales*, Geneva: UNAIDS.

—— (2001) *Drug Abuse and HIV/AIDS Lessons Learned: Case Studies Booklet Central and Eastern Europe and the Central Asian States*, Geneva: UNAIDS.

—— (2003) *Report on the Global HIV/AIDS Epidemic*, Geneva: UNAIDS.

—— (2004a) *Report on the Global HIV/AIDS Epidemic*, Geneva: UNAIDS.

—— (2004b) *The changing HIV/AIDS epidemic in Europe and Central Asia. Joint United Nations Programme on HIV/AIDS*, Geneva: UNAIDS.

—— (2005) *AIDS Epidemic Update*, Geneva: UNAIDS.

—— (2006) *Report on the Global AIDS Epidemic*, www.unaids.org/en/HIV_data/2006GlobalReport/default.asp.

UNAIDS / Open Society Institute (2001) 'Drugs, AIDS, and Harm Reduction: How to Slow the HIV Epidemic in Eastern Europe and the Former Soviet Union', report (New York).

UNAIDS / WHO (1998) *Report on the Global HIV/AIDS Epidemic*, Geneva: UNAIDS / WHO.

—— (2001) *EPI-2001. Report on the Global HIV/AIDS Epidemic*, Geneva: UNAIDS / WHO.

United Nations Development Programme (UNDP) (1994) *Human Development Report*, New York: UNDP.

—— (1995a) *Human Development Report*, New York: UNDP.

—— (1995b) *Public Sector Management, Governance, and Sustainable Human Development: a Discussion Paper*, New York: UNDP.

—— (1996) *Human Development Report*, New York: UNDP.

—— (1997a) *Human Development Report*, New York: UNDP.

—— (1997b) *La gouvernance et le développement humain durable*, New York: UNDP.

—— (1997c) *Reconceptualizing Governance: Discussion Paper 2*, New York: UNDP.

—— (1998a) *Human Development Report*, New York: UNDP.

—— (1998b) *Sustainable Human Development. From Concept to Operation: a Guide for the Practitioner*, New York: UNDP.

—— (1999a) *Central Asia 2010. Prospects for Human Development*, New York: UNDP.

—— (1999b) *Human Development Report*, New York: UNDP.

—— (2000) *Human Development Report*, New York: UNDP.

—— (2001) *Human Development Report*, New York: UNDP.

—— (2002) *Human Development Report*, New York: UNDP.

—— (2003) *Human Development Report*, New York: UNDP.

—— (2004) *Human Development Report*, New York: UNDP.

—— (2005) *Human Development Report*, New York: UNDP

UNICEF (1991) *Structural Adjustment with a Human Face*, Geneva: UNICEF.

UNODC (2002) 'Illicit Drugs Situation in the Region Neighbouring Afghanistan and the Response of ODCCP', report: unpublished.

—— (2005a) 'HIV/AIDS midpoint estimates' report: unpublished.

—— (2005b) 'The Opium Economy in Afghanistan. An International Problem', report: unpublished.

UNODC Regional Office for Central Asia (2003a) 'Organized Crime in Central Asia', report: unpublished.

—— (2003b) 'Global Illicit Drug Trends', report: unpublished.

—— (2004) 'Tajik-Afghan Border Assessment Mission', report: unpublished.

Urjewwick, C. (1993) 'Le Caucase et la Transcaucasie', in M. Ferro and M.-H. Mandrillon (eds) *L'état de toutes les Russies. Les États et les nations de l'ex-URSS*, Paris: La Découverte / IMESCO.

Vidal, L. (2004) *Ritualités, santé et sida en Afrique. Pour une anthropologie du singulier*, Paris: Karthala-IRD.

Visser, A. P., Pavlenko, I., Remmenick, L. and Bruyniks, P. (1993) 'Contraceptive Practice and Attitudes in Former Soviet Women', *Advanced Contraception*, 9: 13–23.

Wedel, J. (1995) 'US Aid to Central and Eastern Europe, 1990–94: An Analysis of Aid Models and Responses', in J. P. Hardt and R. F. Kaufman (eds) *East-Central European Economies in Transition*, New York: M. E. Sharpe.

—— (1996) 'Aid and reform in the former second world', in S. W. Hook (ed.) *Foreign Aid toward the Millennium*, Boulder, CO: Lynne Rienner.

—— (1998) *Collision and Collusion. The Strange Case of Western Aid to Eastern Europe 1989–1998*, New York: St. Martin's Press.

—— (2003) 'Clans, Cliques, and Captured States: Rethinking Transition in Central and Eastern Europe and the Former Soviet Union', *Journal of International Development*, 15: 427–40.

Wedel, J. R. and Creed, G. (1997) 'Second thoughts from the second world: interpreting aid in post-communist Eastern Europe', *Human Organization*, 56(3): 253–64.

Weiss, T. G. and Gordenker, L. (1996) *NGOs, the UN and Global Governance*, London: Lynne Rienner.

Werner, C. (1998) 'Household networks and the security of mutual indebtedness in rural Kazakhstan', *Central Asian Survey*, 17(4): 597–612.

Werth, N. (1992) *Histoire de l'Union soviétique: de l'Empire russe à la communauté des États indépendants,1900–1991*, Paris: PUF.

—— (1993) 'De la soviétologie', *Le débat*, 77: 126–44.

Westhoff, W., Klein, K., McDermott, R. J., Schmidt, W. D. and Holcomb, D. R. (1996) 'Sexual Risk Taking by Muscovite Youth Attending School', *Journal of School Health*, 66(3): 102–4.

Williams, C. (1995) *AIDS in Post-Communist Russia and its Successor States*, Avebury: Gower House.

World Bank (1989) *Sub-Saharan Africa: from Crisis to Sustainable Growth*, Washington, DC: World Bank.

—— (1992) *Governance and Development*, Washington, DC: World Bank.

—— (2005) *Combating HIV/AIDS in Europe and Central Asia*, Washington, DC: World Bank.

World Commission on Environment and Development (WCED) (1987) 'Our common future', also known as the 'Brundtland Report', New York: World Commission on Environment and Development.

Word Health Organization (WHO) (1993) *The Public Health Rationale against Mandatory Testing*, Geneva: WHO.

—— (1995a) 'The Work of the Global Programme on AIDS in Europe: 1994–95', report: unpublished.

—— (1995b) 'TASO Uganda: the Inside Story, Participatory Evaluation of HIV/AIDS Counselling, Medical and Social Services 1993–94', report: unpublished.

—— (1995c) *Global Prevalence and Incidence of Selected Curable Sexually Transmitted Diseases: Overview and Estimates*, Geneva: WHO.

—— (2000) *Report on the AIDS Epidemic Update*, Geneva: WHO.

—— (2001) *Report on the AIDS Epidemic Update*, Geneva: WHO.

—— (2002) *Report on the AIDS Epidemic Update*, Geneva: WHO.

—— (2003) *Report on the AIDS Epidemic Update*, Geneva: WHO.

—— (2004) *Report on the AIDS Epidemic Update*, Geneva: WHO.

—— (2005) *Report on the AIDS Epidemic Update*, Geneva: WHO.

Yoon, S., Shimizu, M., Gedik, G., Falkingham, J. and Pomfret, R. (1999) 'Initial conditions at the start of transition', in *Central Asia 2010: Prospects for Human Development*, New York: UNDP.

Young, A. (1976) 'Some Implications of Medical Beliefs and Practices for Social Anthropology', *American Anthropologist*, 78: 5–24.

—— (1981) 'When Rational Men Fall Sick: an Inquiry into Some Assumptions Made by Medical Anthropologists', *Culture, Medicine and Psychiatry*, 5: 317–35.

—— (1982) 'The Anthropologies of Illness and Sickness', *Annual Review of Anthropology*, 11: 257–85.

—— (1995) *The Harmony of Illusion. Inventing Post-Traumatic Disorder*, Princeton, NJ: Princeton University Press.

—— (1996) 'A Description of how Ideology Shapes Knowledge of a Mental Disorder (Post-Traumatic Stress Disorder)', in S. Lindenbaum and M. Lock (eds) *Knowledge, Power and Practice: the Anthropology of Medicine and Every Day Life*, Berkeley, CA: University of California Press.

Index